Live. Laugh. Smile. Myths and Truths About Today's
Orthodontics and How to Prepare for Your Child's Smile
© 2019 Dr. Valerie Minor, Dr. Brad Mokris

ISBN: 978-1-970095-09-8

TABLE OF CONTENTS

FOREWORD
An Orthodontic Practice -
Talk About Breaking the Mold!

Dr. Brad Mokris, is often asked how he ended up becoming an orthodontist. Truth be told, he will tell you it wasn't his first choice of career paths. In kindergarten, his teacher asked the class what they wanted to be when they grew up. Confidently, Dr. Mokris stood up and told the class he wanted to be an astronaut. That was, though, until his friend whispered in his ear, "Sometimes when astronauts go up in space, they get lost and don't come back down." Needless to say, he never sent his application in to NASA. He did, however, have the experience of getting braces in high school, and after finishing treatment he spent many hours shadowing his, and other, orthodontists throughout high school and college. Dr. Mokris knew from that very early stage in life that this was his "perfect" career. He is extremely proud and appreciative of what he gets to do every day.

"I create smiles...what a job!" – Brad Mokris

After college, and a not so brief hiatus surfing in Hawaii, he spent 7 years in Gainesville, Florida receiving his dental and orthodontic training. It was there that he feels fortunate to have met the one and only love of his life, Jennifer, also a dentist practicing in Fernandina Beach. They have 4 children - Avery, Reese, Austin and Graham. Aside from their careers, the children are their life, keeping them on their toes endlessly. Orthodontics is a constantly evolving and exciting field. At Coastline Orthodontics, Brad and all of the doctors he works with truly believe that they have an obligation to provide their patients with the safest and most advanced treatment options available.

"This is not something that is learned once but an ongoing learning process with continuing education and a lifelong pursuit to be the best at what I do. These aspirations help me to give my patients individualized treatment geared for the most healthy and efficient path towards a beautiful smile."
–Brad Mokris

Dr. Valerie Minor, an orthodontist at Coastline Orthodontics recalls not always wanting to be an orthodontist either. After doing a 9th grade science project on "Which toothpaste whitens the best?" she did consider dentistry as a career choice. However, when it was time to go off to college, she could not imagine going to school for another 8+ years, so instead, she decided to get an engineering degree. After graduating from North Carolina State University with degrees in Chemical Engineering and Pulp and Paper Science, she was fortunate to get a great job working as an engineer for Rayonier in Fernandina Beach, FL, near her hometown.

After a short time working in the manufacturing industry, Dr. Minor decided that this was not for her. But, as luck would have it, while working at Rayonier, she spent some time shadowing Dr. Suellen Rodeffer in her orthodontic practice. She realized very quickly that this was a profession that she would love. Why? Well, to Dr. Minor it seemed to combine the engineering that she had learned with the interaction and care for people that she was missing in a manufacturing facility. She was amazed to see the changes that would take place and the smiles on the faces of Dr. Rodeffer's patients when they would leave her office. In fact, Dr. Rodeffer actually joked with her that one day she would come back and be one of the partners in the practice. Little did Dr. Minor know that God was planning that very path for her.

With the blessing of her husband, Dr. Valerie Minor made up her mind to pursue that very goal. After taking several prerequisite courses while still working for Rayonier, they packed up and moved to Gainesville, Florida for 7 years of training at the University of Florida. Dr. Minor has never regretted one second of that decision and will tell you to this day how much she loves her career and how grateful she is to be practicing with such amazing mentors. She joined the husband/wife team of Rodeffer and Garner Orthodontics in 2006, and her husband, Will, was able to teach and start the baseball program at the newly opened Yulee High School. The practice then became Rodeffer, Garner, and Minor Orthodontics shortly thereafter, and now they have changed the name again to Coastline Orthodontics with the addition of Dr. Mokris to the practice. Dr. Minor and her husband have 4 amazing children named Harper, Savannah, Ava, and Addison (twins). Needless to say, the kids keep them very busy, but they are the joy of their lives.

Drs. Brad Mokris and Valerie Minor are two of the four owners/orthodontists at Coastline Orthodontics. They have offices in Jacksonville, Fernandina Beach, and Macclenny, FL. They provide orthodontic treatment to patients all the way from North Florida to South Georgia and beyond. It is the hope of both Dr. Mokris and Dr. Minor that every patient, new and old, will feel comfortable in their practice, and they appreciate the trust that everyone places in them.

The doctors sincerely enjoy getting to know each and every patient and they love watching the transformation that takes place as patients develop more confidence in their smiles.

If you were to ask any of the orthodontists at Coastline what is unique about their practice, they would emphatically state that it is the fact that they are a privately owned 4-doctor, 4-location practice. So, why is this important? There are many benefits, which are often overlooked. The #1 benefit is that each one of the doctors has ownership in the practice, which in essence means that there is an extremely high level of patient commitment and patient-centered relevance surrounding the decisions that are made in the practice.

Secondly, consistency among the doctors is a crucial element in achieving good orthodontic outcomes. Since all 4 of the doctors are invested in the practice (and are not just employees), they have reason to make sure that every single individual patient's treatment plan is executed in a way that maximizes the chance of achieving the best possible results.

The doctors at Coastline Orthodontics are continuously striving to make their practice work for them. They are, in fact, constantly working to decrease expenses, increase efficiencies, improve customer service, and expand the array of dental services they provide. This practice has very special owners who are fixated on their commitment to success. They are repeatedly involved in advanced, forward-thinking training and consider their practice to be exclusive. They do whatever it takes to sustain that exclusivity and are determined to be the best of the best.

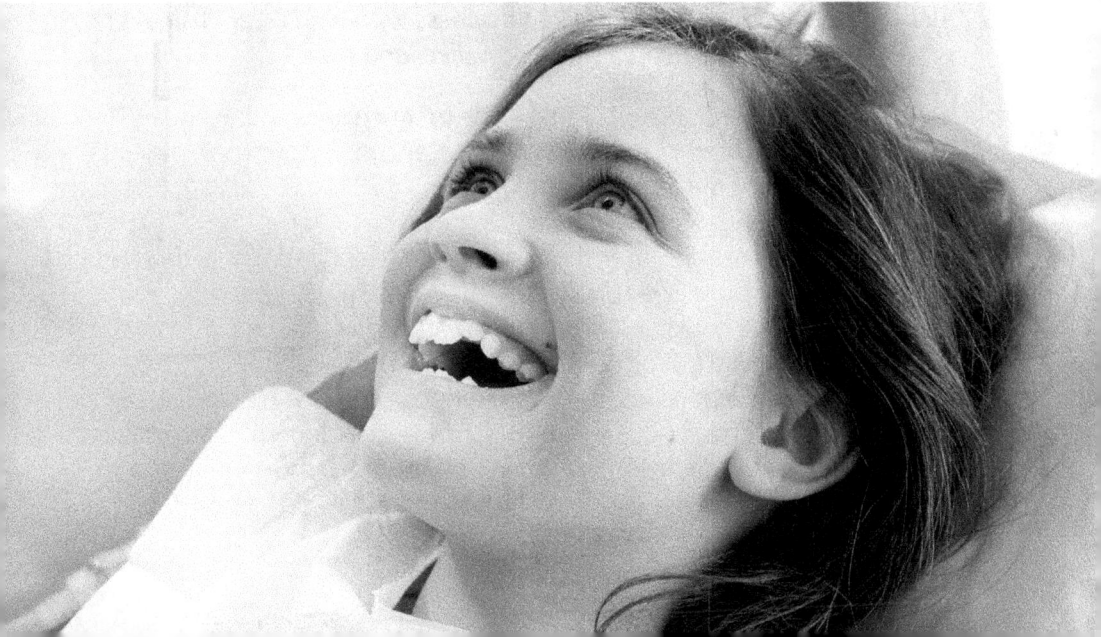

Do they have a secret to delivering great customer service? Yes, actually, they make it their #1 priority to serve their patients and their families. It's not about filling the schedule, it's not about making more money, but rather it's about treating people the right way. They believe that if you follow that philosophy, everything else will fall in place, and it does!

Here are some ways that Coastline Orthodontics delivers great customer service:

They Recognize the Value of Word-Of-Mouth Referrals – Great word-of-mouth referrals are a priceless asset for any practice. These doctors really focus on and value the things that positive word of mouth does for the practice which is one reason that their patients fall in love with them.

They Design Their Patients' Experience – They make sure the customer experience is nothing short of delightful, and immediately start building customer loyalty.

They Manage Patient Expectations – They learn immediately what the customer expects, ask open-ended questions and understand the patient's perception. They listen and accept feedback and are thorough and honest. And most importantly, they communicate well and often.

"All things being equal people will do business with, and refer business to, those people they know, like, and trust."

They Treat Their Patients Like Royalty – The practice knows that their business depends on how well and how consistently they put their patients' needs at the forefront of everything they do.

The #1 reason that parents refer their family and friends to this orthodontic practice is trust – bottom line. It's a given that every family coming into this office is looking for a beautiful smile. Not only is it the responsibility of the practice to provide that, but also, in their opinion, it is the minimum they should be providing. Expertise is expected when you go to a specialist's office, and that expertise stems from a combination of factors including experience, education, continuing education, and clinical skill. The orthodontists at Coastline more than cover their bases in those categories. However, first and foremost, the main reason people refer to their practice is truly trust. It is one thing to be a good orthodontist, it is a completely different thing to be a good human being. Ask one of these doctors and they will tell you:

> *"We are good people. We take care of our patients and our team members, and we see that commitment reflected throughout our referring patients and colleagues."*

After all, we all share a responsibility to contribute to a more truthful, authentic world where folks can trust the providers in their lives. The doctors appreciate this authority because they have unique experiences, stories, insights, and information to share with their patients. You may not trust a friend who makes claims about orthodontic procedures, but when you speak with a trusted authority who is credible, you are far more likely to take the information seriously.

Aristotle held that 3 characteristics are essential of the authority in question in order to generate an atmosphere of trust:
- the character of the speaker
- reliability and honesty
- and the goodwill of the speaker.

One of the biggest reasons that Dr. Mokris, Dr. Minor and the entire practice have done so well is their ability to build that much-needed trust. They hold themselves to honesty as a nonnegotiable standard, and they keep their promises.

The entire team at Coastline Orthodontics can easily be described as family, plain and simple. They continuously treat each other as such and make it a point to welcome each and every patient to become a part of that family. With 4 doctors and 20+ team members, they have plenty of family love to share, and they pride themselves on welcoming new patients and team members to the club!

Do you feel that you are an important part of your healthcare provider's practice? It's important that you do. In fact, as the customer, you are the most important part of the family. As orthodontists, and the owners of their practice, these specialists engage their clients with compassion and make them feel appreciated and respected. By listening intently and communicating efficiently with patients, they are better able to develop a treatment plan precisely around their needs. Team members, patients and their families are the center and most valuable part of the team. The doctors involve the patients in their own care and recognize that they are the most essential part of the practice. They encourage their patients to be proponents of their own care and let them know that it is okay to ask questions and to take charge of their plan.

Continuing Education

Orthodontics is a science, and just like science, it changes as new information is learned through research. This makes it vital for orthodontists to always continue their education to stay on top of the latest developments. And, not only is it important (and required by law), but Dr. Mokris and Dr. Minor believe it to be even more increasingly significant in today's rapidly changing environment. And, not all continuing education is equal. Therefore, they try to maximize their attention in multiple areas of the orthodontic atmosphere, but definitely focus heavily on patient satisfaction and clinical advances with technology.

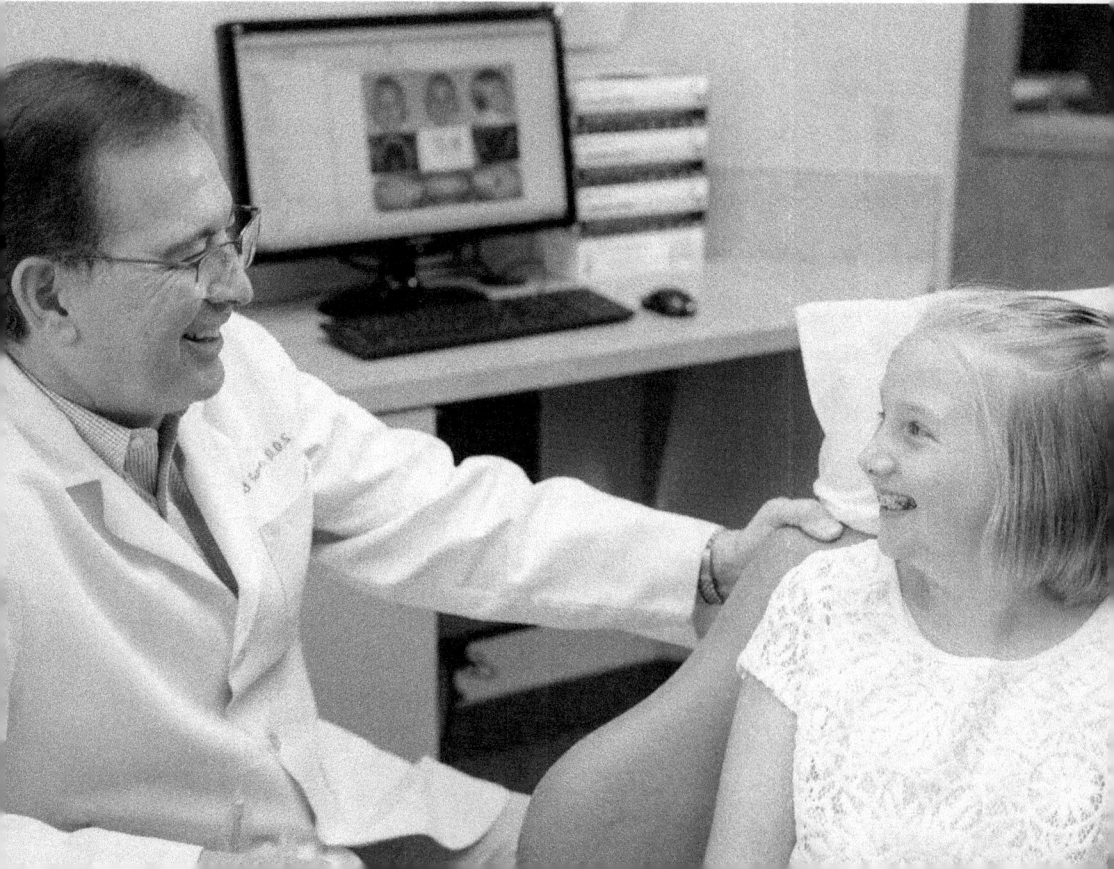

The methods, tools, and technologies of orthodontics tend to change even faster than the theories behind them. Even in a few years, new technologies develop, leaving old treatments outdated and no longer used. Only by attending seminars and taking further classes can orthodontists learn about these cutting-edge new treatments. While the Coastline doctors are proud of the level of expertise that they offer their patients, don't expect them to brag about their credentials during appointments. In fact, quite the contrary. Dr. Mokris and Dr. Minor alike are known for being outgoing, welcoming, friendly, and very resourceful. Your appointments will be fast, relaxed, and fun! The energies of Dr. Mokris and Dr. Minor and their team members to produce an office setting that combines expertise with fun makes your orthodontic treatment exceptional and pleasant.

Mentoring

Drs. Mokris and Minor have both had two significant mentors in their careers. Their current partners and the founding orthodontists of the practice – Dr. Suellen Rodeffer and Dr. Tod Garner, who have both been a great inspiration in many ways. A wonderful, married couple, they have taught so much over the years. They continue to be great advisers, not only at the orthodontic and business level, but also at a personal level. Drs. Rodeffer and Garner are generous, caring people who do so much for their community without wanting any recognition. In addition, the practice is always open to welcoming mentees, who have consisted mostly of middle school, high school and college students who are interested in, or currently pursuing, a career in the dental field.

Here's the bottom line - At Coastline Orthodontics, the doctors believe that the best thing about their practice is their patient family. Period. They will tell you that they are nothing without their patients. Therefore, they are continually striving to show their appreciation.

A favorite quote:

> **"To whom much is given, much is required."**
> Luke 12:48

Drs. Mokris and Minor feel honored and blessed to have been given the opportunity to change people's lives through orthodontics. The art and science of orthodontics is a big responsibility. The doctors understand this and are committed to providing the patients and families of Coastline Orthodontics with superb customer service and beautiful smiles.

In conclusion, Dr. Brad Mokris and Dr. Valerie Minor both bring extensive operational experience in orthodontics to this private practice and are committed to excellence. They are keenly focused on the needs of their patients and driving a culture that always puts their patients first above all else.

They are dedicated to dispelling the stigma associated with issues regarding trust in the orthodontist/dentist because of a lack of understanding about how dentistry works. Feel free to contact either doctor with questions at www.coastlineorthodontics.com.

Call us at 904.600.4749 or go to www.coastlineorthodontics.com to schedule your own Customized Smile Analysis.

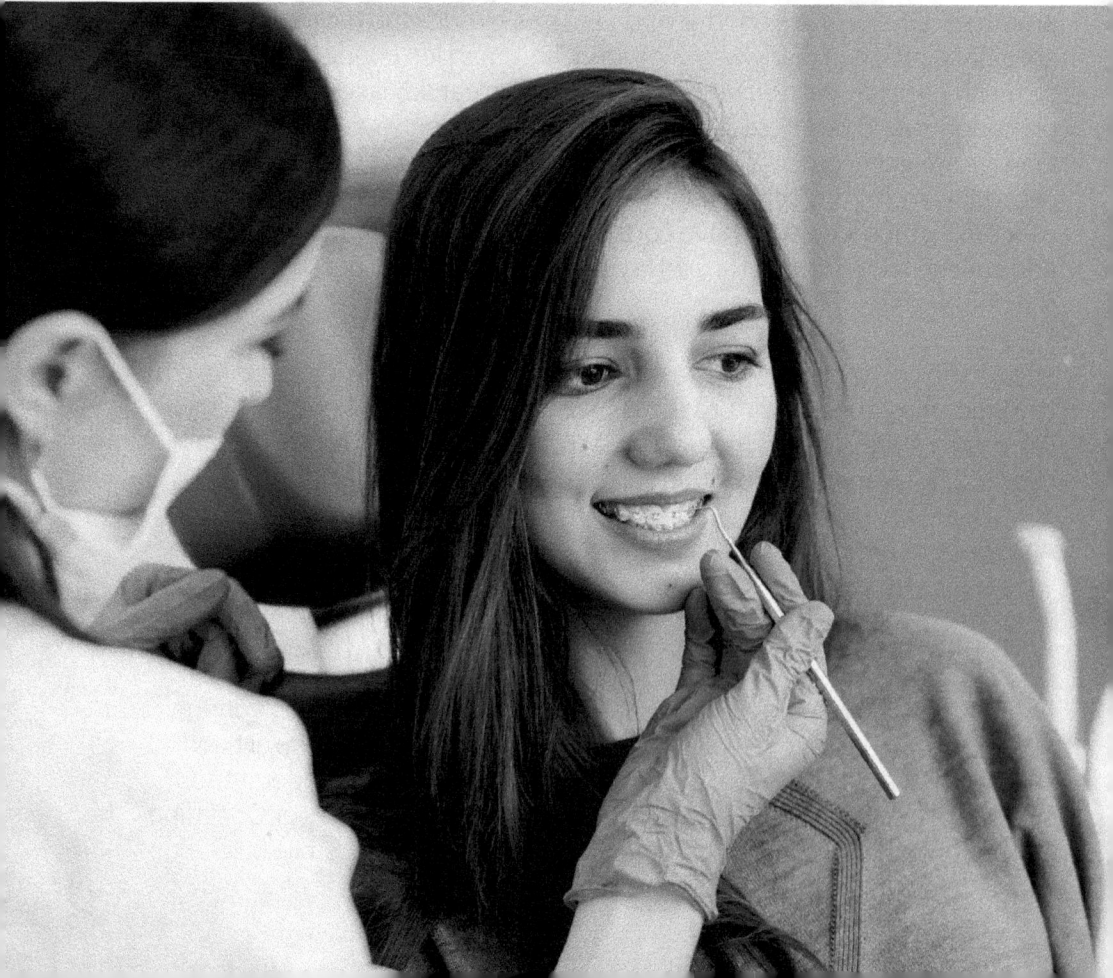

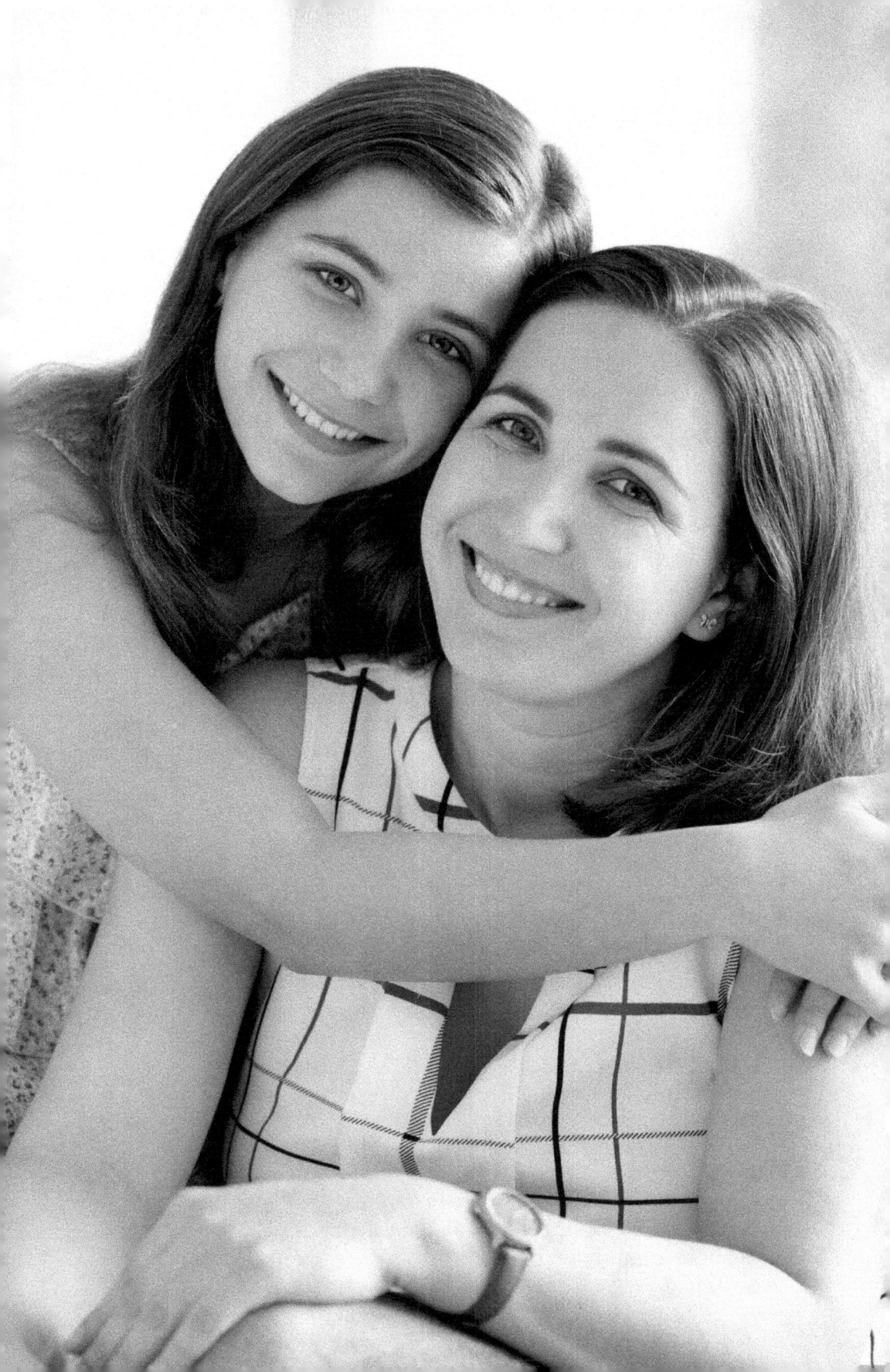

CHAPTER 1

Why is My Child's Smile So Important?

If you are weighing the yes/no and now/later decisions of orthodontic care or braces, you'll be trying to decide just how important or unimportant it really is.

Some parents feel "looks aren't everything." Some think their kid should just be tough-minded about this and not overly sensitive. Some may not have had orthodontic care when they were children and think, *Hey, I turned out just fine. I have a great spouse, a good career, friends—so what's the big deal?*

But that was then. This is *now*: the age of social media.

Social shaming and bullying is a lot worse, a lot more common, and a lot more persistent than when you were a kid. Teen suicide is on the rise, and such suicides share one thing in common: shocked and bewildered parents who could not conceive of their child ending his own life. Sure, they might've noticed he was a *little* depressed. They knew he was being bullied and spending more time home, alone, not leaving his room, but geez, he *is* a teenager, after all. What once was a few days or weeks of misery contained in the cafeteria with a few bullies is now endless, expansive, and broadcast online to everybody. Behind a computer screen, it can get far nastier than most would dare in person. Sometimes, kids bully each other for no reason. Being a "buck-toothed" girl or a boy with gaps in between the teeth can sometimes be enough to exacerbate the situation.

Signs Your Child May Be Being Bullied

- Decrease in self-esteem
- Not wanting to go to school
- Skipping school
- Injuries they can't explain
- Self-destructive behaviors (e.g., harming themselves)
- Declining school grades
- Sleep difficulties
- Loss of interest in schoolwork or activities
- Sudden loss of friends or avoiding social groups
- Changes in eating habits

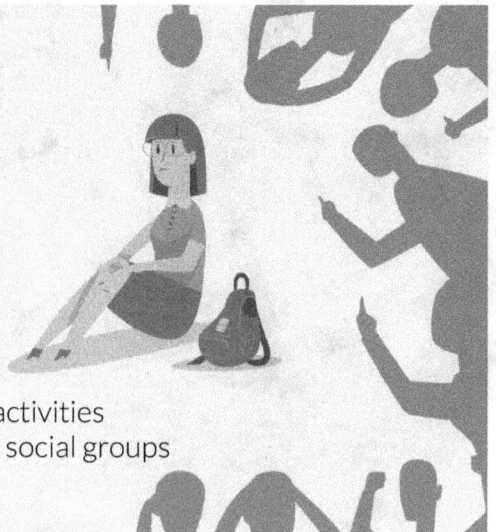

A straight, clean and healthy smile can not only give your child the confidence needed to embrace true worth, but can also pave the way toward easier socialization at school, church, or during extracurricular activities. Do your child a favor and talk about their smile and how it might be affecting them.

Beyond that, there's a life ahead of your child. Going to middle school with crooked teeth and a smile that you're not proud of is one thing. Hey, plenty of kids are going to school *without shoes* for heaven's sake. But going to college admission interviews, packing up and heading off to college, going to job interviews, trying to fit into new and anxiety-rich environments at a faraway college or new workplace with a smile that you're not proud of is more serious.

This isn't *just* a cosmetic issue. Misaligned, crooked teeth can contribute to *significant* medical problems.

Poorly aligned teeth or a poor bite can contribute to chronic headaches and migraines, contribute to digestive problems because of the inability to properly chew foods, and make getting a decent night's sleep impossible. Maybe most dangerous of all, it can foster gum disease. Gum disease has absolute links to diabetes, heart disease, strokes and dementia, as well as, of course, the loss of natural teeth altogether. Orthodontic corrections can be done later in adult life but often they can be more difficult. We treat a large number of adult patients at Coastline Orthodontics, and most of them say they wish they would have had treatment earlier in life.

Mouth problems and misaligned teeth that are not corrected could cause problems with your gums and the bones that support your teeth. This could allow "pockets" for infections and periodontal disease to arise and turn into very difficult, painful and costly problems later in life.

In the teenage years, failure to spend even $ 4,000 can easily create a $40,000 full mouth restoration case at age forty or fifty or embarrassing, health-compromising removal of all teeth and use of dentures at age sixty.

Gum disease is serious business. It worsens the risks of and heightens dangers from diabetes, heart disease, strokes, and dementia. Ignoring teeth misalignment in pre-teen or teen years could lead to adult medical problems. If there is a genetic history of any of these medical problems, you only worsen the odds of your son or daughter suffering from them by ignoring or postponing needed orthodontic treatment.

Aside from impacting health, a poorly aligned smile can significantly impact your child's comfort. Headaches, toothaches, sinus problems, dry mouth, snoring, drooling, bad breath, and insomnia are potential symptoms of a smile that isn't straight, jaws that aren't aligned, or teeth that are too close together or not quite close enough. Oftentimes, however, the mouth is the last place we check for signs of discomfort, loss of sleep, or even a simple headache.

If your child's pediatrician can't figure out why they're not sleeping well or why they're experiencing headaches or even insomnia for which there seems to be no cause, a simple thirty-minute exam at your local orthodontist could provide a clear solution in no time!

This is what we hear from a lot of adult patients getting orthodontic treatment and braces:

> *"I had wonderful parents,* **but** *they could not afford the braces I needed. I wish I had gotten the care I needed when I was a kid, so I didn't grow up to have this smile my whole life* and have all these problems now."

All parents want to do the right thing. They don't want to let their children down in any way. Parents just about kill themselves over their kids' college, trying their best to guide the decision, trekking around the country on campus visits, worrying over campus culture, or taking on *serious* debt. Every parent understands what many kids can't—that it's not about the few years of college but rather the forty or fifty years afterward.

The same thing applies here. An investment in orthodontic treatment now would provide immeasurable benefits over the years to come. Kids can't always appreciate that now, but you can.

No parent wants their child to suffer, either from teeth that actually hurt, headaches you can't explain, insomnia that affects their daily life, or insecurity your child may be feeling because of a crooked or oversized smile.

The fact is, your child's formative years are actually the most sensitive for his or her teeth. Now is the time to pay close attention to your child's smile, behavior, peer relationships, and confidence level.

If any or all are lacking, a qualified orthodontist may help give you and your child the peace of mind you both crave.

The Top 5 Reasons People Avoid Seeing the Orthodontist

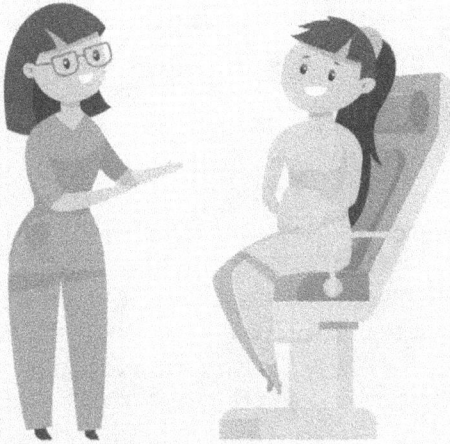

1. Patients are afraid it's going to hurt.

Pain is the number-one reason most people avoid going to the orthodontist. However, modern technology—and choosing the right orthodontist—can ensure that your child enjoys his/her orthodontic experience with minimal discomfort.

2. Patients are afraid it's going to cost too much.

Not only are most orthodontic procedures more affordable than ever, but insurance, payment plans and a variety of other financing options make this all but a moot point for most of our patients. Remember, orthodontists are here to make sure your child's teeth, smile, and jaw are aligned to make his or her life better—period! We're not going to let something like price get in the way of creating a better, safer, healthier smile for your child.

3. Patients are afraid it's going to take too long / miss too much school or work.
Regardless of the type of orthodontic procedure your child needs, time is of the essence. Modern technology and ease of access allows us to work around your child's school schedule with minimal absences. After initial visits, and barring the actual procedure itself, most visits and/or adjustments are routine and can take anywhere from fifteen to forty-five minutes.

4. Patients do not see the need to take action. Eroding, crooked or unaligned smiles can take time to happen, but the time to act is now. Orthodontic irregularities don't just heal on their own or disappear if you ignore them. Your child's smile and overall dental health are too important to ignore out of questions of pain, convenience, or even price.

5. Patients have been treated in the past with an attitude of indifference. Let's face it, not all doctors are created equal. There is no room for indifference when it comes to your child's healthcare. Find an orthodontic specialist that offers not only state of the art technology for your child but state of the art service as well. Orthodontic specialists know what it's like to sit in the chair, and should provide every opportunity for patients, especially our younger patients, to feel comfortable, safe, and secure in our care.

Call us at **904.600.4749** or go to www.coastlineorthodontics.com to schedule your own **Customized Smile Analysis.**

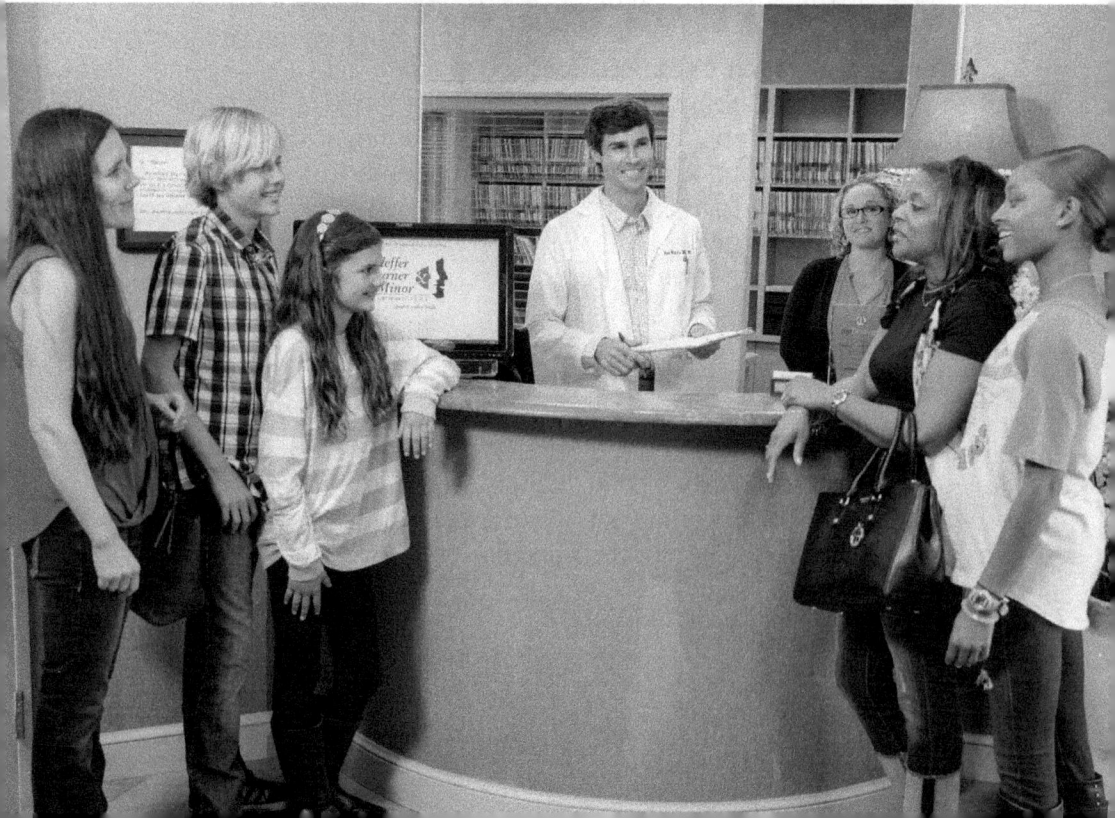

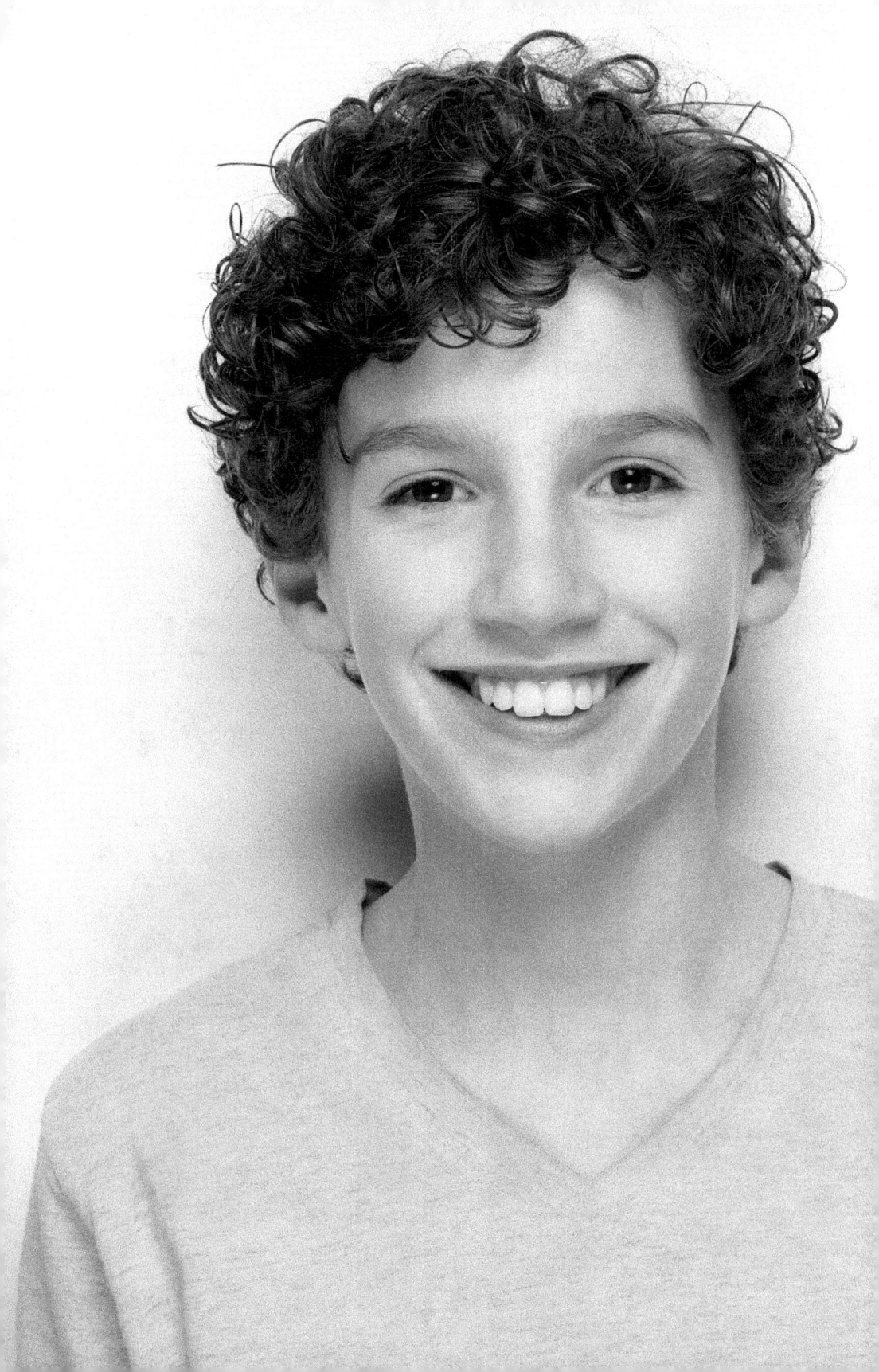

CHAPTER 2
Why Do Kids Need Braces?

Are braces something created by orthodontists to make money, like Disney figured out with the extra-charge FastPass? Was it a conspiracy from the very start?

There may be some overprescribing and premature prescribing by some doctors. There are bad apples in every orchard. And you know the adage: if all he's got is a hammer, everything (and everybody) looks like a nail.

There is a very legitimate, clinically documented, and often a clearly visible reason why some kids, as young as eight, *need* orthodontic treatment and care: malocclusion.

Malocclusion is mostly genetic, so if your daughter or son has it, blame their grandparents. It's a fancy-pants term for all things related to misaligned teeth; teeth growing angled, crooked, and into a space that's too small. It can be a single tooth, a few teeth, or the whole mouth. As I said, it is mostly hereditary, but there can be other causes too, like premature loss of primary teeth, chronic thumb-sucking, or even an accident that seemed to leave no lasting effect at its moment in time.

If your child is suffering from any, several, or all of the following early indicators of malocclusion, consider having them addressed by an orthodontic specialist sooner rather than later:

- **Crossbites:** A crossbite occurs when the jaw deviates to one side with an improper fit of the upper and lower teeth from left to right or front to back. Crossbites can lead to worn and chipped teeth, jaw pain and asymmetric growth of the jaws. Left untreated, the crossbite will require more extensive treatment later in life and significant jaw surgery in the most-severe cases.

- **Thumb-sucking:** Thumb-sucking habits that continue after at age seven should be corrected immediately in order to prevent severe jaw and tooth alignment problems.

- **Miscellaneous concerns:** There are several other issues you should also be looking for as soon as your child turns seven in order to intervene early. These include the following:

    - Permanent teeth that are growing into the wrong spots
    - Severely protruded front teeth at risk for injury or causing teasing at school
    - Severe crowding with permanent teeth erupting into poor-quality gum tissue

With any of these situations, we can discuss the pros and cons of early intervention and treatment versus waiting until all the permanent teeth are in for braces. If you are anxious about the appearance of your child's teeth or your child is self-conscious about his or her appearance, early treatment might be the best choice. Not only are most orthodontic problems more difficult to correct later, but self-image and personality inhibition can be hard for a person to leave behind. However, if your child is extremely resistant to braces or is not mature enough to be trusted to care for them, delay may be the better choice. In that case, regularly scheduled orthodontic check-ups will be necessary.

Having malocclusion does *not* guarantee a child will need braces. Frankly, this is what worries me about nonspecialists like family dentists substituting themselves for orthodontists, and parents letting it happen. They may easily miss an early diagnosis of malocclusion, when it could have been averted without braces. Or they may leap to braces as the only way to treat all malocclusion. Either way, you and your child lose.

The first question, then, is: does your daughter or son have or show any of the signs they are going to have malocclusion? If so, what—of numerous options—should be done about it? When?

To have all these questions answered early, the first full orthodontic exam should occur early in a child's life. We recommend seven or eight, no later than nine, especially if there is family history of malocclusion. With early and periodic exams by an orthodontic specialist, you may avoid his need for braces and/or you may prevent years of suffering and embarrassment related to his teeth and smile.

Waiting could have serious consequences, often requiring more treatment and higher costs later in life. What most parents fail to realize is that these problems are urgent and should be treated as such. If that ship has sailed, the next best time for a full orthodontic exam is tomorrow!

Fun Fact: At Coastline Orthodontics, the doctors usually recommend early treatment to only about 10% of children. If your child is one of those of 10%, pat yourself on the back for bringing them early and saving them from all sorts of problems that could have occurred if you had waited.

If your son or daughter does need braces—now or at some predictable future time—the outcome of the exam can lead to *sensible* decisions. If not now, treatment to prevent the need could begin, or your could begin saving money for braces or other procedures that may be necessary later on in your child's life. There is no tooth fairy coming to leave a few thousand dollars underneath a pillow of yours. But if the need must be met three years from now, skipping one Starbucks run a week for those three years can make a hefty dent in the bill to come. Utilizing a Health Savings Account or Flex Spending Account can help, as well. Later in the book, we discuss how to fund orthodontic treatment.

Let us be emphatically clear. We are *not* in the business of putting braces on any child who doesn't need braces. Our office is *not* a braces store. We are in the business of helping kids and families get this right: get the right orthodontic treatment if any is needed, get the right braces if any are needed, and have as perfect a smile and as few oral health problems as possible. We make sure our patients are informed—that's why we wrote this book. You're provided with real information, no medical jargon, plain English, "reasons why" and options.

Kids do need braces, but not all kids and certainly not the same braces for all. Some kids are better served by other orthodontic treatments instead of or before braces. We will collaborate to figure out what is or isn't needed and what options are best if there is a need for your child.

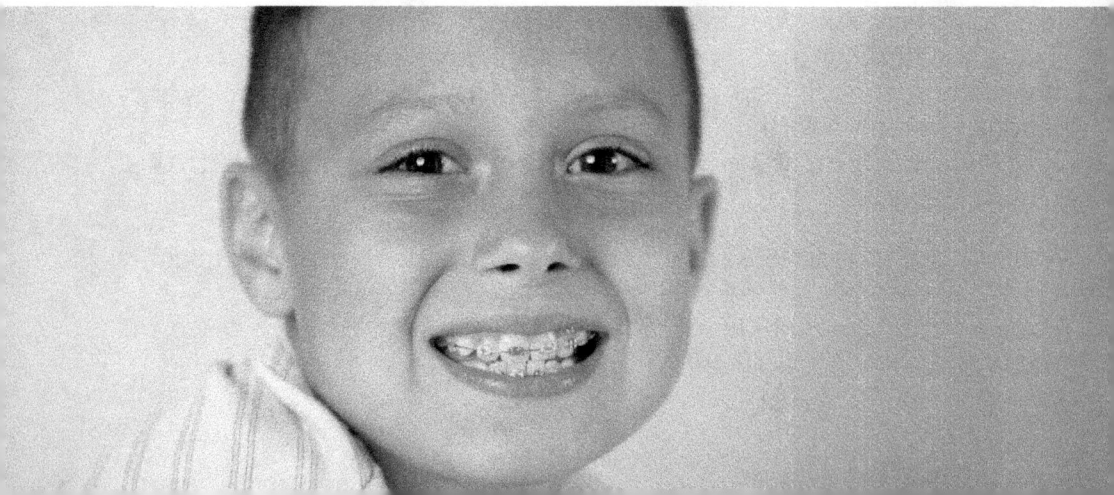

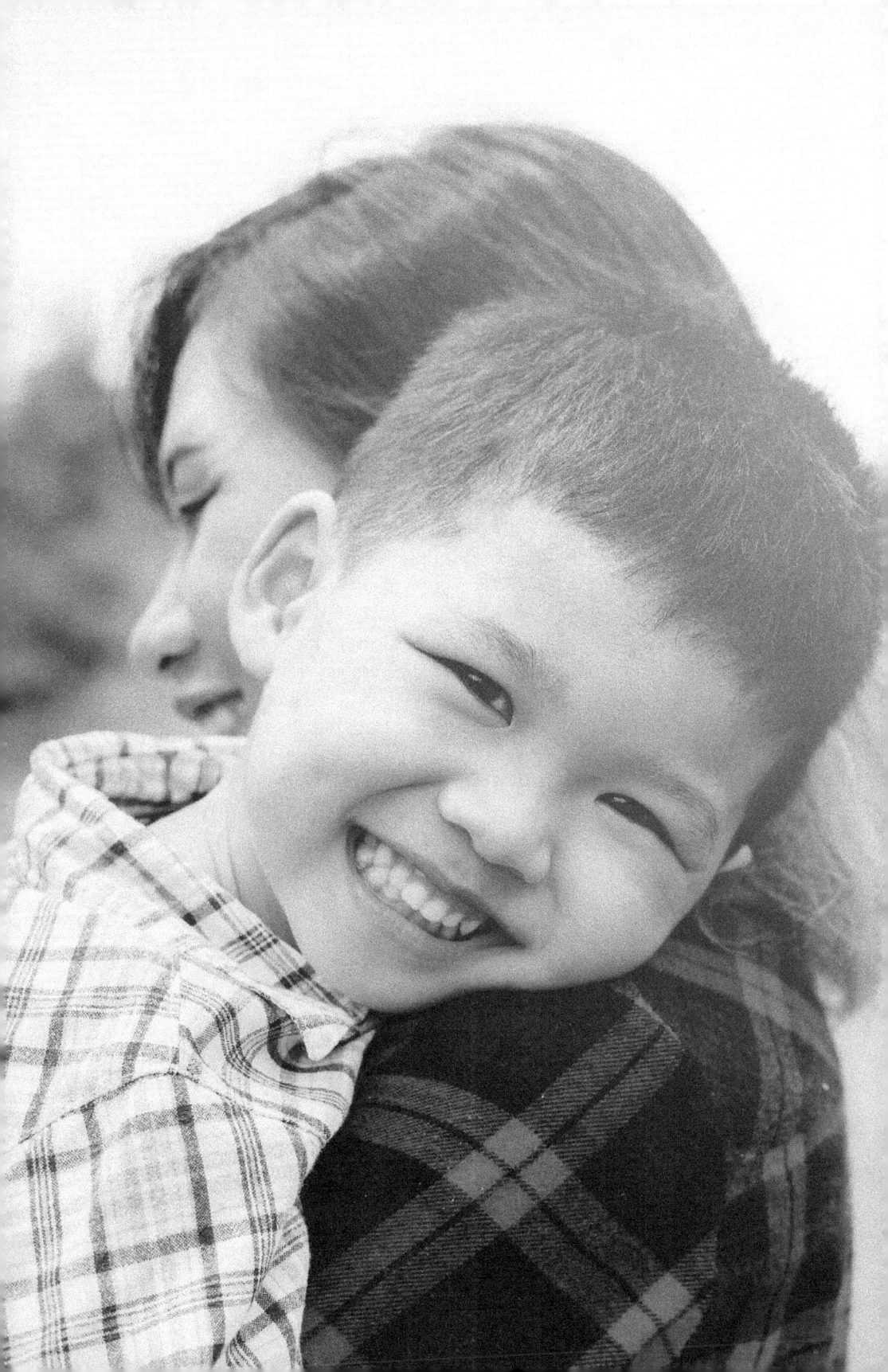

CHAPTER 3

Why Not Just a Dentist? Why an Orthodontist?

You undoubtedly already have a dentist.

Gee, isn't seeing an orthodontist going to cost a lot more?

I'm busy. More appointments?

Do I really need to get orthodontic check-ups for my kids? My dentist didn't mention that we needed one.

Don't worry, these are all reasonable questions! It is true that, today, quite a few dentists dance over into our territory, and although they're not permitted to claim they're the same as orthodontists, they're able to do things like provide Invisalign and braces. This can be confusing. Here are the facts.

All orthodontists are dentists and we all graduate from the same dental schools. True enough. But that's where it stops for dentists. Orthodontists go to school for an additional two to three years to become credentialed specialists at diagnosing and providing the best treatment for conditions like:

- Difficulties chewing or biting
- Constant biting into the cheek, gums, or roof of the mouth
- Teeth that meet abnormally or don't meet at all
- Teeth grinding or clenching
- Crowded, misplaced or blocked out teeth
- Early or late loss of teeth
- Teeth growing in poor positions
- Teeth that protrude
- Embarrassing personal appearance due to teeth
- Facial imbalances
- Teeth or jaw misalignment, TMJ
- Chronic headaches and migraine
- Poor sleep
- Speech difficulties (that may never be outgrown or may develop later)

These are not dental care issues. They are orthodontic issues.

For *some* things, a generalist will do. For other things, you know it's smart to seek out the best specialist you can afford. For example, if all your income is in a single W-2 from one employer and you have simple, ordinary deductions, getting your taxes prepared for the cheapest fee at the seasonal H&R Block office that opens up in your neighborhood shopping center is probably fine. But if you have W-2, 1099 and investment income from real estate, depreciation on real estate in several states, own stocks and you raise iguanas as a money hobby, you're going to get yourself a really good accountant, probably a CPA.

If you need the simplest will, leaving everything first to spouse or second to daughter may be okay. But if you are of some means and have several children and maybe also grandchildren as well as charities, you're going to need to see an *estate planning attorney*: not just any attorney. They all went to the same law schools—but you would need a *specialist in estate planning*.

This is no different.

There are a few things to keep in mind when differentiating between a general dentist and an orthodontic specialist.

First, generalists often work with one-size-fits-all, off-the-rack, standardized solutions. They may be limited to doing only what the computer dictates that they do, without bringing expertise and expert judgment to bear. They're often working with products from only one provider, without being able to select from a full range of options that would work best for you. Specialists, instead, tend to individually and carefully diagnose needs and provide personalized solutions.

Second, generalists and their use of standardized solutions tend to be cheaper than the fees of a specialist, but that also places economic pressure on them to do the treatment as quickly and simply as possible.

In this case, it's worth remembering that the treatment provided has permanent, lifelong, and life-impacting consequences. This concerns your health. Future dental or jaw alignment or misalignment issues can affect quality of sleep (which can affect weight, even onset and management of type 2 diabetes and heart disease), as well as self-esteem and social and career success.

General Dentist. A general dentist gives routine checkups, preventative measures, cleans teeth, and fixes cavities. They may not start seeing children until they are seven to ten years old.

Pediatric Dentist. A pediatric dentist has two to three years of specialized education beyond dental school. They specialize in providing dental care to children and adolescents, typically from first tooth to age 18 offering checkups, preventative measures, cleanings, and filling cavities.

Orthodontist. An orthodontist has two to three years of specialized education beyond dental school and is an expert at straightening teeth and aligning the jaws. They assess patients and determine the best treatment route to straighten their teeth and align their jaws.

If you can, you want to choose an orthodontist for orthodontic care.

You may ask, *how do I know my doctor is an orthodontist?* It's a good question and a critical one to ask as you seek additional treatment for your child's dental issues.

Only orthodontists can belong to the American Association of Orthodontists (AAO). If you're looking for a local orthodontist, go online and visit **www.braces.org** to find a specialist in your area. This website features not only a searchable database of orthodontists but educational tips, answers and resources to help you on your quest for your child's healthiest smile!

Alternatively, you can ask your doctor if he or she has completed a two- to three-year residency in orthodontics and check with your state dental board to follow up on his reply. Dentists and orthodontists in most states will be registered differently with the dental board.

Do your homework; be a "dental detective" while on the hunt for such vital information. Look for the words "dental specialist in orthodontics" or ask your general dentist for a referral to a specialist. In urban and suburban areas, it will take minimal effort to find a specialist. In more remote, rural locations, your search might take you to another city or town. Don't be afraid to ask your dentist if an orthodontist travels to your town every month to see patients. There's a chance an orthodontist from a larger city comes to your town and works out of another dental office once or twice per month. Looking around can save valuable driving time and money.

One note: there is no disrespect between orthodontists and dentists. As a matter of fact, many orthodontic patients are referred by their dentists. These are great, capable, and caring professionals who know where their expertise begins and ends, and they do not let ego or income opportunity step in front of what they know is best for their patients. Dr. Mokris understands this personally and professionally. He is married to a dentist. Just as the family doctor refers his patients with possible or significant heart disease issues to a cardiologist, and if need be, the cardiologist refers to a cardiac surgeon, the best dentists refer patients with orthodontic needs to orthodontists. Orthodontists are required to take two to three extra years of university education beyond dental school and additional continuing clinical education every year. They must also invest in state-of-the-art technology for their offices (not found in dental offices) —*all for a good reason*.

Even though we orthodontists have the education and training to perform general dentist procedures, we don't. We specialize.

Call us at 904.600.4749 or go to www.coastlineorthodontics.com to schedule your own Customized Smile Analysis.

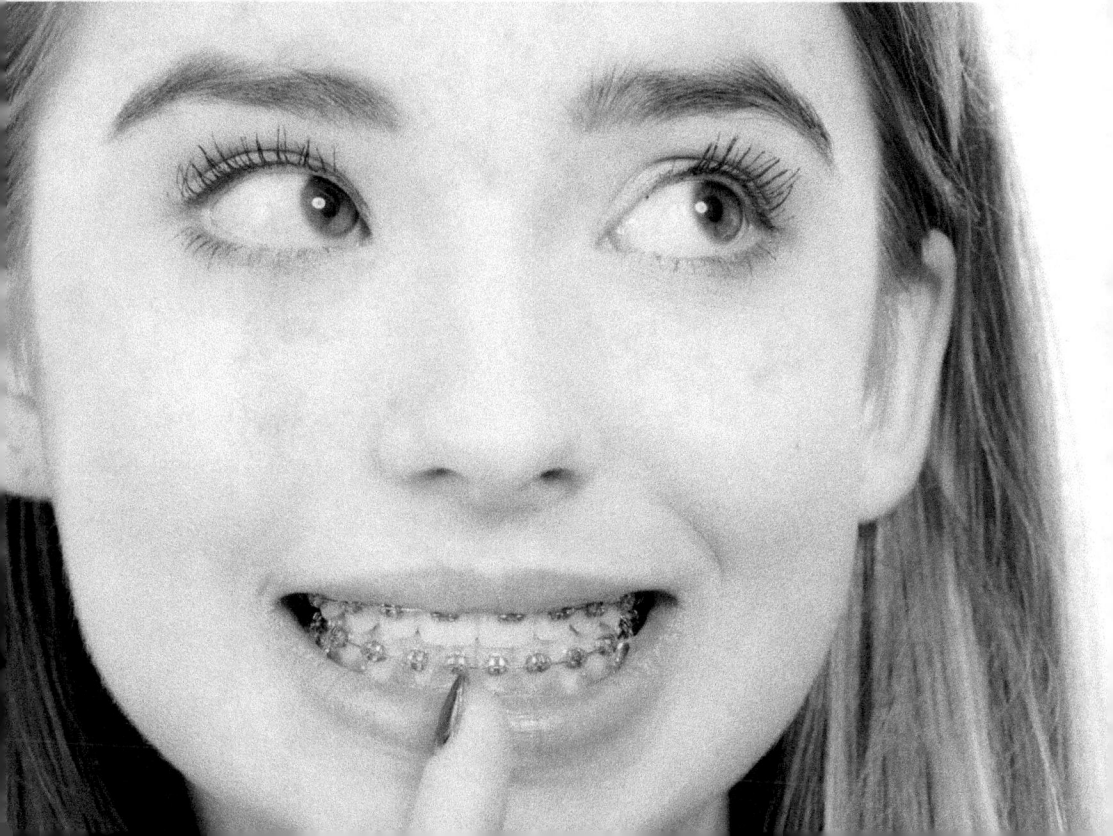

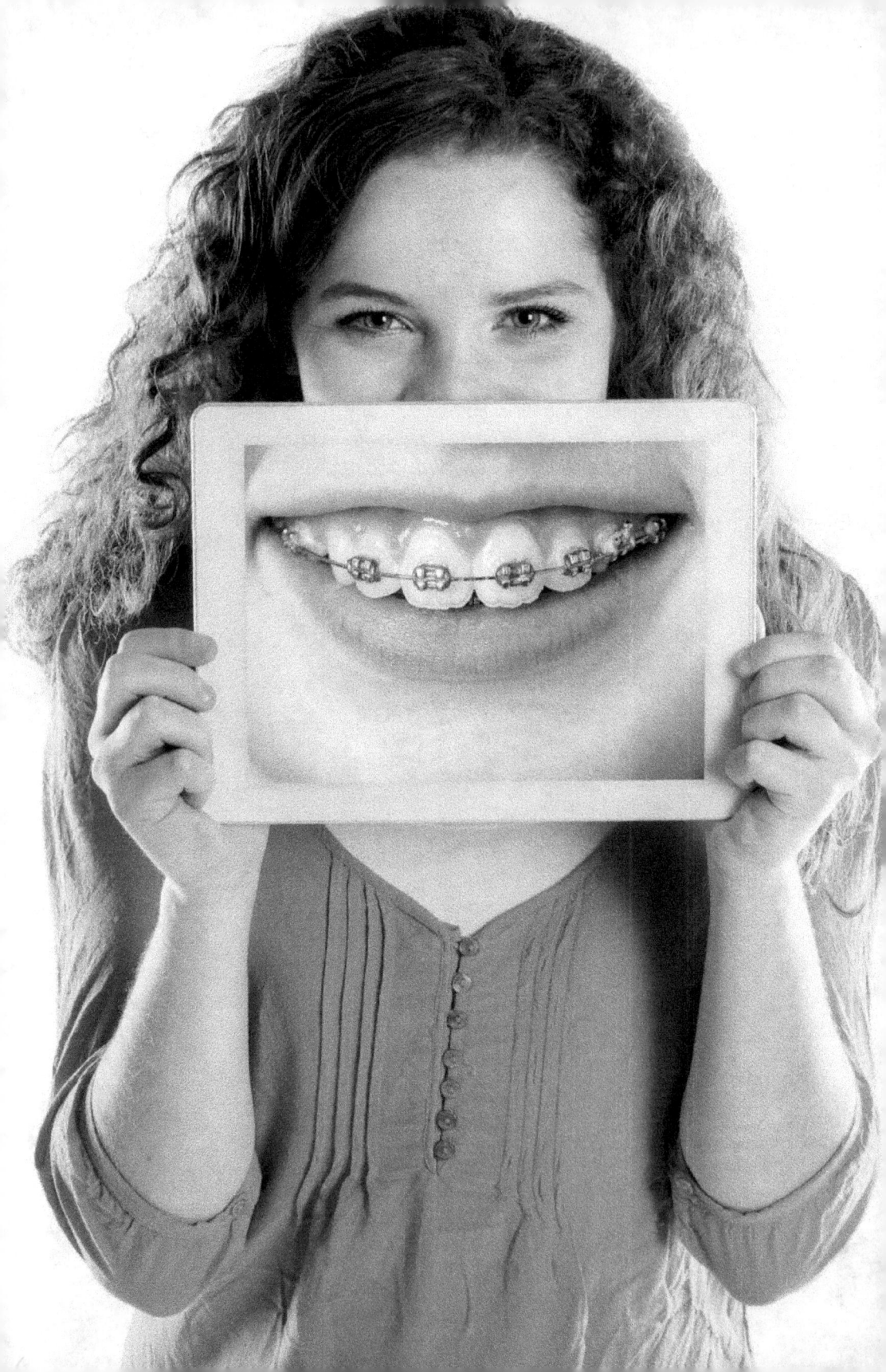

CHAPTER 4

Choose a Highly Successful Orthodontist

Why is that important? Wouldn't you get a "better deal" from one barely getting the light bill paid? Maybe. But an overeager orthodontist—or maybe more so, an overeager dentist wanting to do braces—might be seeing needs that are more urgent than they really are.

What are some good clues to selecting a great orthodontist?

I've got two: One, He's busy. His practice is busy.

I assure you, the ability of advertising to attract orthodontic patients is limited and it's expensive. When you see a really, really busy practice, there are probably a whole lot of patient referrals. Kids and parents would not enthusiastically refer if they felt they were lied to or treated badly, put in pain or wound up with results nothing like the digital future-photo they were shown. And they probably wouldn't recommend the practice if they had to keep coming back to "fix a few things," or were overcharged. Parents tell parents about great orthodontic practices because we earned their trust and because their kids keep thanking them.

We keep our office busy. Yes, we advertise. But mostly, orthodontic practices thrive by patient referrals. Not that we would anyway, but we don't need to goad you into more or more expensive care than your son's or daughter's situation requires for the best outcome. We don't need to "sell" four more sets of braces this month to win a cruise from the manufacturer—and yes, that stuff goes on in some practices. There's an old cartoon from The Wall Street Journal with a bunch of executives in a boardroom at a conference table, one hollering, "Ethics? Ethics? We can't afford ethics!"

This is a business, a business built on ethics and earned trust. And you do not just need a doctor to install braces; you need a trustworthy, trusted advisor.

The other clue: a great orthodontist is *not* cheap.

Our fees are calculated to allow for quality care in every respect, to put no downward financial pressure on how we care for patients and parents, and to never cut corners or take shortcuts. We never use any material that is "probably good enough."

If I were you, I'd worry if I could find an orthodontist that is a lot cheaper than anywhere else. If you do find one, know this: behind closed doors they're probably asking, "Can we do this cheaper?" Is that the question you want discussed back there, at every step of your child's treatment?

This isn't even like Botox. It's more like cosmetic surgery. There's a science and an art to this. Our orthodontists and our staff are all highly trained to produce state-of-the-art outcomes, nothing less. The doctor makes a difference. That's why we tell everybody to get a highly successful orthodontist.

The Top Ten Things You Should Know *Before* Choosing Your Orthodontist

This is something you want to be sure about. I've just suggested one big consideration: a very successful practice. Here are nine more.

1. **Are they specialists?**
   As previously discussed, orthodontists are specially trained dentists who take on several extra years of training in order to "straighten teeth," usually by affixing braces to the patient's teeth. You might say we specialize in smiles. Orthodontists also perform dentofacial orthopedics. This is a fancy way to describe how we normalize the structure of a patient's jawbones in order to repair any imbalance in their face. All orthodontists are dentists, but only 6 percent of dentists are orthodontists. Look for the seal of the American Association of Orthodontists (AAO). Only orthodontic specialists can belong to the AAO.

2. **Do they treat adults?**
   Orthodontics is not just for kids! It's important that your orthodontist can treat patients of all ages. Many adults are finding out how a healthy and attractive smile is important to their health and the way they feel about themselves. Others choose to avoid a lifetime of crooked teeth for health concerns or problems with their bite.

3. **Do they provide the first visit free of charge?**
   Most orthodontists offer complimentary examinations for new patients so you and your family can get expert advice about treatment needs, options, and timing before making this important investment. During your first exam and consultation be sure your questions are answered, your concerns are addressed, and you are educated about all of your treatment options.

4. **Are they using the latest technology and treatment options available?**
   Orthodontics today differs a great deal from years past. Specially designed braces and wires dramatically increase the precision with which we move teeth and shorten treatment time. Tie-free braces systems are sometimes used to make treatment more efficient. Clear braces offer a cosmetically pleasing alternative, while Invisalign offers patients an entirely brace-free option. Did you know that Invisalign also has a special treatment system just for teens?

5. **Does their quoted fee include retainers?**
   Each orthodontic office has its own fee schedules, and doctors often charge differently for procedures. All orthodontists should offer you a contract that clearly spells out the expenses for your child's treatment before it begins.

   Throughout the orthodontic industry, it's common to find out about retainer fees after you start treatment. You should ask your orthodontist about what retainers cost and also if there are any other hidden fees.

6. **Do they charge for "comfort visits"?**
   Some minor discomfort may occur with braces. Orthodontists typically provide adjustments for poking wires and loose appliances free of charge. At Coastline, we do provide these types of adjustments free of charge, but you should definitely ask about adjustments and potential costs with your orthodontist before you start treatment.

   Keep in mind; if your braces are broken or damaged due to noncompliance with dietary restrictions, this may result in repair charges. With Coastline Orthodontics, if you do your best to avoid breaking your braces and follow the simple dietary guidelines that we will share with you, then you should have no additional costs for adjustments throughout your treatment, even if something is broken.

7. **Do they make you feel special and comfortable?**
   Regardless if you are reading this book for your own treatment or for your child's treatment, when you meet with your orthodontist, you should definitely feel comfortable. At Coastline Orthodontics, we strive to make you as comfortable as possible before, during, and after treatment. You are special and we want you to feel that way every time you see us. Particularly important if you are reading this book for the treatment of your child, we also ensure your child feels great every time they visit.

Since our doctors are so involved with children and young adults, we can empathize, relate to them, and make them feel comfortable and extra special.

8. **Do they have a great reputation?**
   With the internet, it is extremely easy to pull up ratings and reviews from patients. Simply go to Google and search for orthodontist reviews and ratings within your town.

   Additionally, look on the website for video testimonials from actual patients. You can also ask the orthodontist for references.

9. **Are they flexible with payment options?**
   Once you are comfortable and you know specifically which orthodontist you want to treat you or your child, the next question is typically, "How much is this going to cost and how am I going to pay for this?"

   We help you understand different payment options from maximizing your insurance benefits to flex spending accounts to even interest-free payment plans. During the initial exam and complimentary consultation, we will answer all of your questions, including those about our typical cost of treatment and the variety of payment options available.

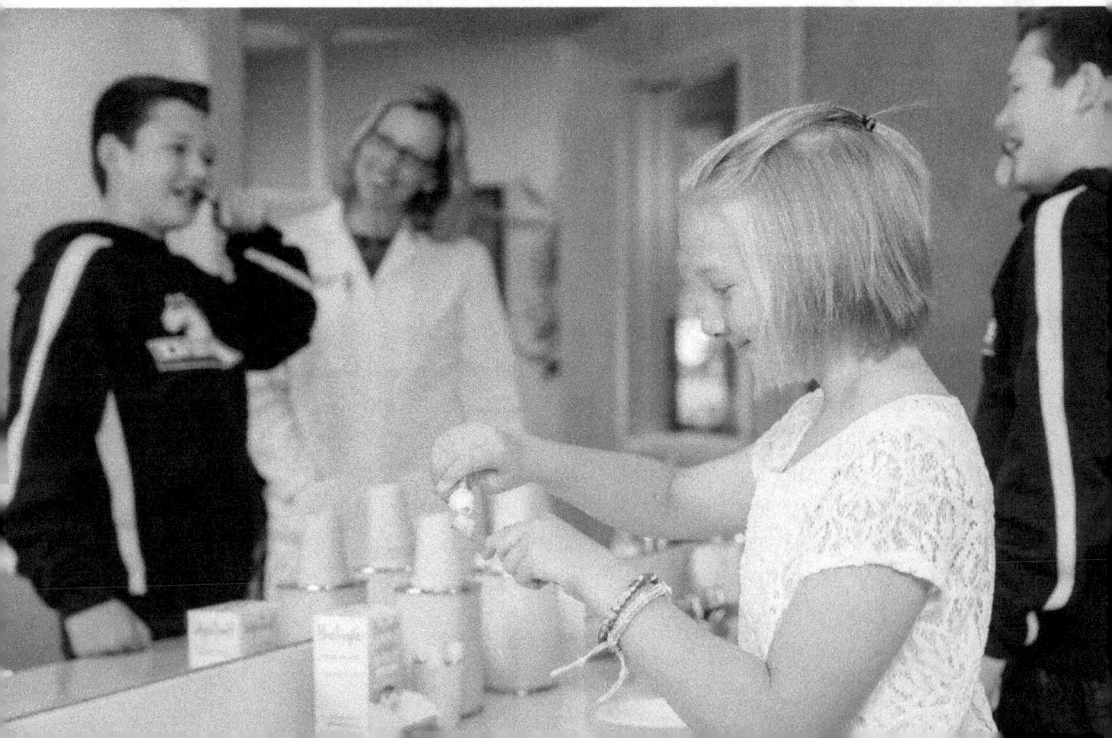

How to Know What Questions to Ask

We've really thought through the questions most parents and patients have—not just the ones they all ask but the ones they don't. This book attempts to cover them all, but overall, this is a personal matter. The best questions to ask are the ones that matter most to you and your child.

We hope not, but you may be in a position absolutely requiring you to get the minimum essential treatment for the lowest cost. If so, your most important questions are going to be about those kinds of options and about price, and about nothing else.

If, however, you are able to make your decision about who you should trust with your child's oral health and smile by many factors, we've included a "What Is Most Important to You?" quiz from Excellence In Orthodontics, on the following pages. As you'll see, there are thirteen different items to consider and rank in importance to you. Any can become the questions you ask us and our team or any other orthodontist.

If you have a specific question not answered anywhere in this book, or have a personal and confidential question, you can—with compete assurance of privacy and courtesy—call our office at any time to discuss you or your child's needs.

There is also a FAQ section at the back of this book.

Of course, a perfect opportunity to get questions answered—yours and your son's or daughter's—is at your exam appointment.

Call us at 904.600.4749 or go to www.coastlineorthodontics.com to schedule your own Customized Smile Analysis.

QUIZ: What Is Most Important to You?

Directions: For each **Key Item** below, rank its importance to you from 1 to 5. Then check off whether each type of provider provides that item. When you're done with all 13 Key Items, add up your rankings and review what your final score means about choosing an orthodontist.

	Key Items to Consider in Selecting Your Orthodontist	Rank How Important Each Item Is To You in Selecting Your Orthodontist 1 - NOT Important, 5 - VERY Important	Check Off If Provided		
			Coastline Orthodontics	Other Provider	Other Provider
1	Orthodontist and staff committed to expert, thorough diagnosis and prescription of the best treatment plan customized for my son or daughter	1 2 3 4 5	✓		
2	Avoiding extractions (if possible)	1 2 3 4 5	✓		
3	Avoiding having to wear headgear with braces (if possible)	1 2 3 4 5	✓		
4	Avoiding "metal-mouth" braces (if possible) or utilizing the new type of "invisible" braces	1 2 3 4 5	✓		
5	Having a healthy, pleasing smile that will last a lifetime and protect optimum dental heath (not just having straightened teeth)	1 2 3 4 5	✓		
6	Treatment with minimal pain	1 2 3 4 5	✓		
7	Orthodontist utilizes the most modern, advanced, and proven technology.	1 2 3 4 5	✓		
8	Orthodontists and team actively involved in continuing clinical education	1 2 3 4 5	✓		

Key Items to Consider in Selecting Your Orthodontist	Rank How Important Each Item Is To You in Selecting Your Orthodontist 1 - NOT Important, 5 - VERY Important	Check Off If Provided		
		Coastline Orthodontics	Other Provider	Other Provider
9 Reducing treatment time to a minimum without compromising results (including total length of treatment term and number of office visits)	1 2 3 4 5	✓		
10 Availability of after-school or after-work appointment options	1 2 3 4 5	✓		
11 Treatment Coordinator is knowledgeable about insurance coverage and is able to offer flexible payment plans	1 2 3 4 5	✓		
12 Getting the best overall value factoring in thorough diagnosis, customized care, and concern with lifetime health and well-being—not just the cheapest fee	1 2 3 4 5	✓		
13 Orthodontist and team committed to excellence in orthodontics and customer service for both patients and parents	1 2 3 4 5	✓		

Total of Your Rankings

What Your Score Means

50 to 65 There is no doubt. Coastline Orthodontics is the right choice for you and your family! It is clear that you place a high value on a comprehensive, "best" approach.

43 to 49 You are probably also going to be happiest with Coastline Orthodontics, rather than any other alternative. But this score suggests you aren't completely sure and have some unanswered questions or concerns. Your doctor and the practice's treatment coordinator want no lingering uncertainties on your part, and want to address any and every question. Don't keep anything to yourself. Please ask.

42 or less Cost may be much more important to you than other factors, or very basic service may be all you feel you need. It's perfectly okay. If you choose to shop around, be sure to use this checklist in evaluating other options. Remember, you do want everything right the first time and you want error-free orthodontics at a minimum.

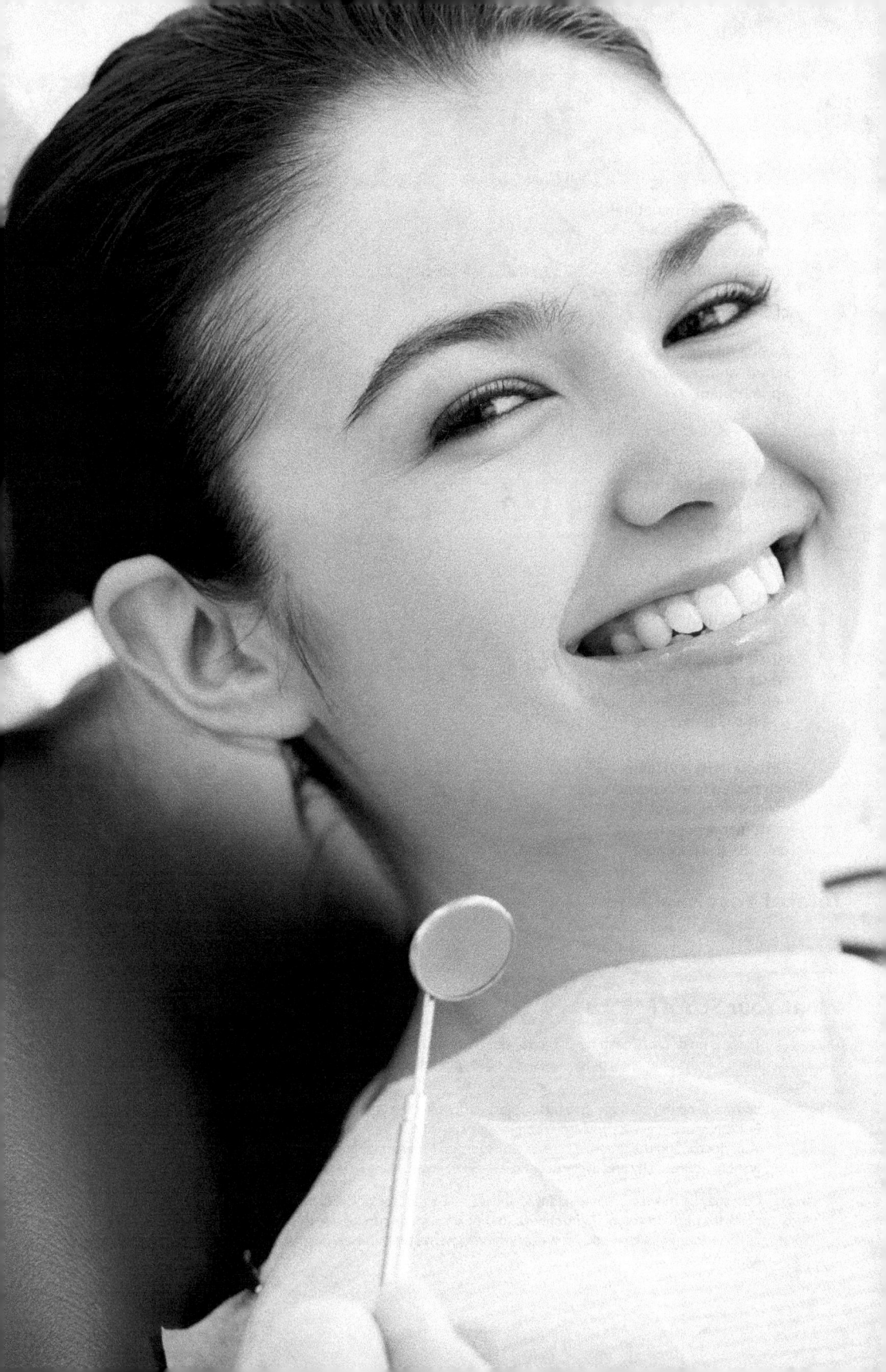

CHAPTER 5

What Can I Expect at the Initial Consultation and Exam?

Many questions surround your first visit to a new orthodontist, not the least of which is the subject of this particular chapter: *what will happen at the initial consultation?*

To answer this very common question, and perhaps several others you might not even realize you need answering yet, let me walk you through the typical first office visit, from the initial appointment forward. Your first appointment is scheduled following your initial phone call to your orthodontist's office.

1: **On arrival at the office, you will be greeted by one of our treatment coordinators.** She or he is fully prepared to make everything from the first appointment to an entire treatment program go smoothly for you and your child. Your treatment coordinator will be yours, to manage your relationship with us, from appointment scheduling for your convenience to answering questions.

At the initial visit, your treatment coordinator will review your child's patient information and health history and and/or any appearance concerns with you.

2: **Next, your orthodontist will conduct the "Customized Smile Analysis,"** the most complete and thorough orthodontic exam, including teeth, gums, mouth, jaws, and face. Typically, safe digital X-rays are taken of the teeth and surrounding bone and of the jaw structures. Molds of the teeth may be made. That same day, your orthodontist will discuss the full state of your child's teeth, gums, mouth and jaws, and diagnosis of any present or anticipated problems. If treatment should be necessary, your orthodontist will present recommendations and options. This will be an individualized, personalized plan of treatment, not "braces in a box, off the shelf."

You will know:

- What teeth or jaw misalignment or other problems exist or are developing

- What the health ramifications are of not intervening with treatment

- What the appearance ramifications are of not intervening with treatment

- If braces are needed now, later, or at all

- Which type of braces will be best in your situation

- What the complete treatment program will consist of: things like braces, number of appointments, and average time of each office visit

- What results will be achieved

3: **All your questions will be answered.** There are no dumb or embarrassing questions. Of the countless patients who have visited our office, every one of them had questions! We do not want you or your son or daughter just nodding, then later wondering, "what did they mean by that?" or saying "I wish I'd asked about ..." This is not one of those "I'm the doctor—trust me—just do what I say because I said so" offices. We know it's a lot to take in. So, any and all questions you have should be asked and answered. Our goal is not just a terrific orthodontic outcome ensuring a healthy, attractive smile but also your anxiety-free comfort from start to finish.

4: **Finally, your treatment coordinator will explain the costs of the prescribed treatment program and discuss payment arrangements as needed.** Presuming that you will be proceeding with treatment, the next appointment will be scheduled, for the installation of braces and/or other treatment. As the saying goes, a journey of a thousand steps begins with the first one, and a task well begun is sooner done!

> *"Our experience with the orthodontist has been better than we ever expected. My son is so proud of his smile, more and more every day."* — Mary C.

In total, you should allow about one hour for this entire initial consultation and exam.

If that seems like a lot, keep in mind that orthodontic treatment could have lasting positive effects on your health, appearance & personality. It is not like "installing tires"—not if it is done properly and expertly. Your son or daughter deserves a careful, thorough, exam that will eliminate anxiety. You want to make the best decisions for them.

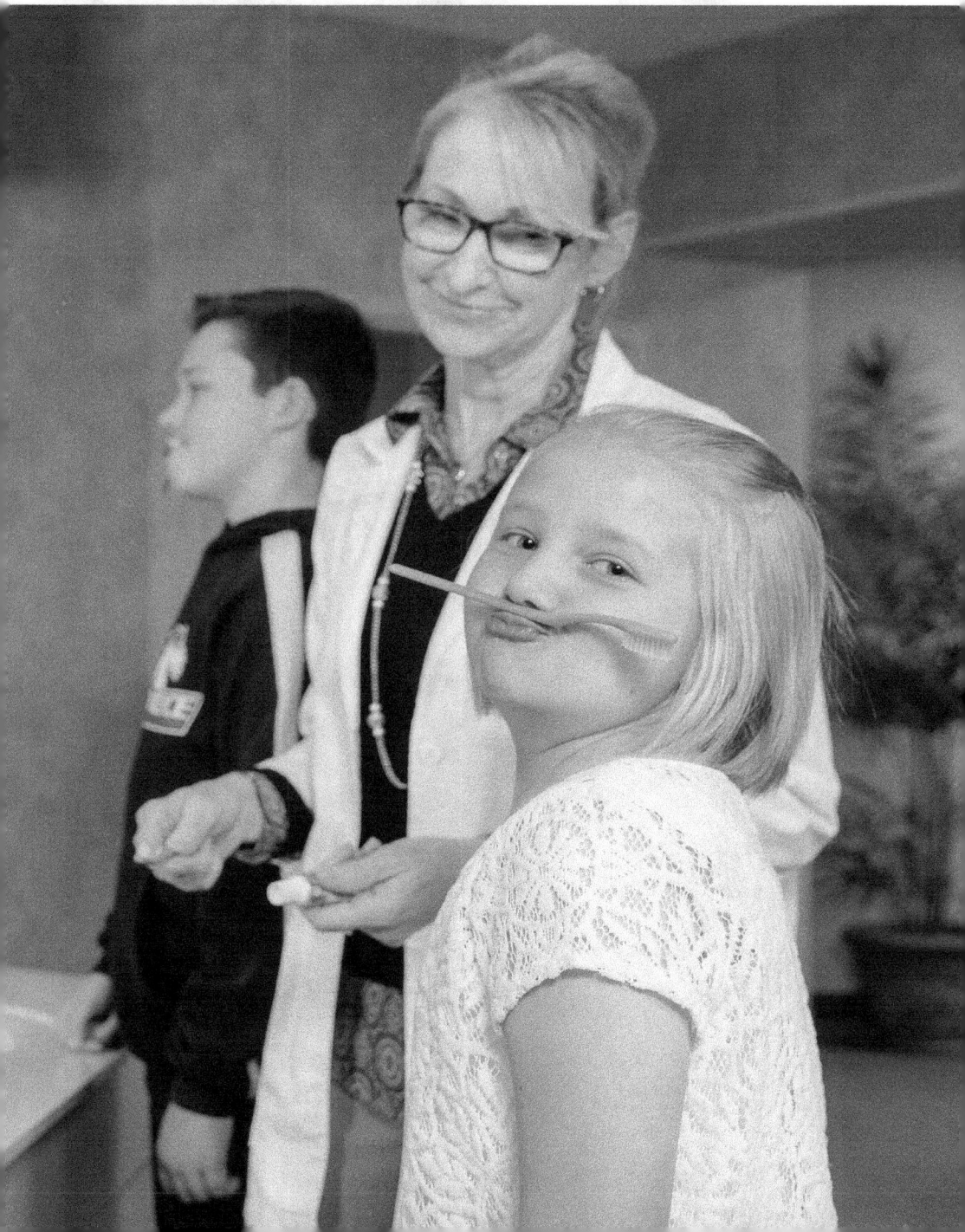

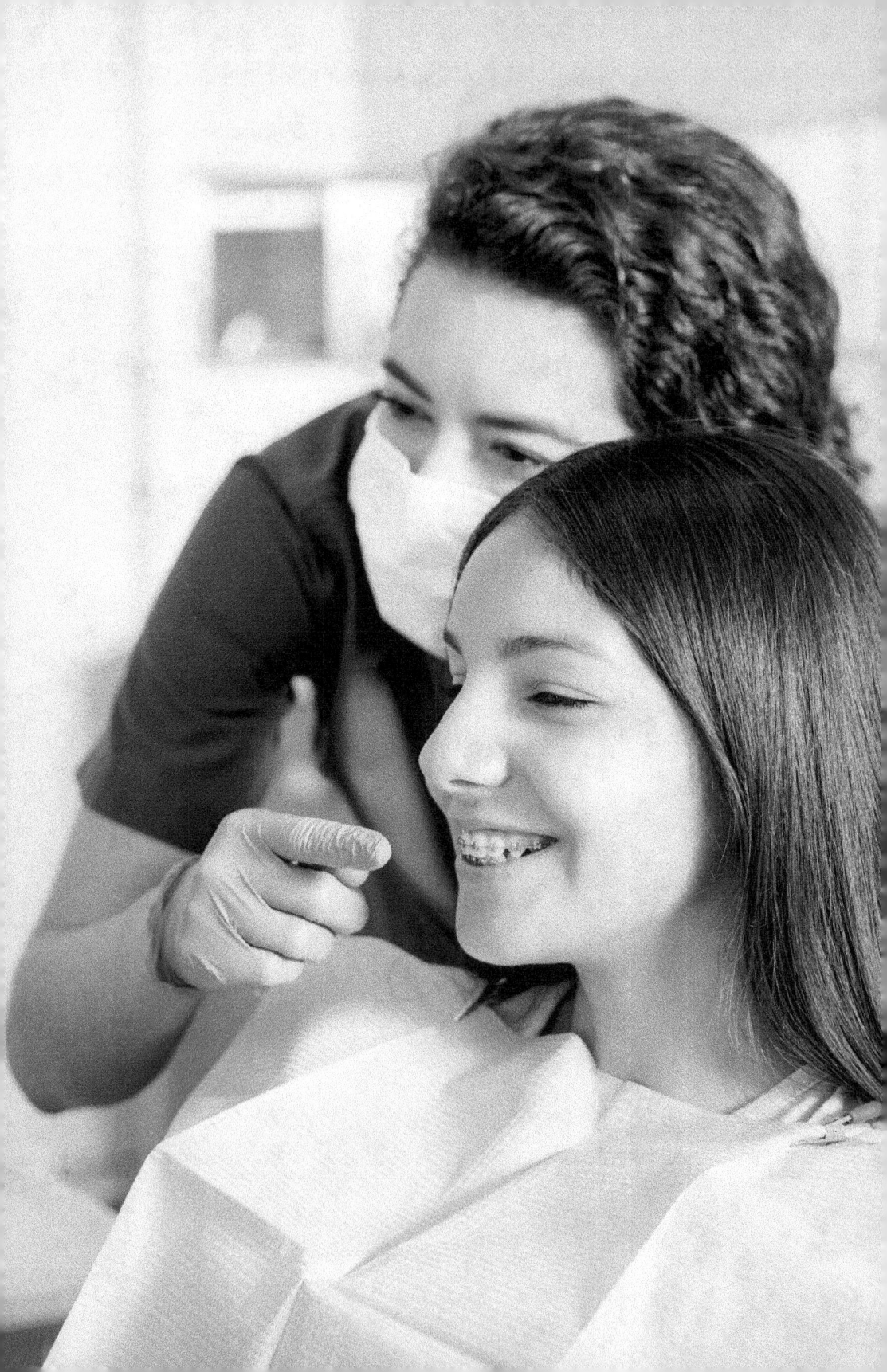

CHAPTER 6

How to Get More Information

There are several ways to get information about an orthodontic practice. First, we want to address the ways we don't recommend.

We don't recommend Yelp. Yelp is, unfortunately, not at all what it seems and is frequently the subject of lawsuits from business owners and under regulatory scrutiny centered around the poorly policed manipulation of reviews and even flooding of fake reviews by "bots" no less! So, beware! Get the information you need from truly trusted sources.

Google can also be deceptive, though I admit it can be a valuable starting point. Rankings are manipulated by advertisements, websites, YouTube content, and what's called SEO, or search engine optimization. The only thing you know for sure about dentists or orthodontists who come up at the top in Google rankings in your community is that they are good at SEO or, more likely, good at paying somebody who is good at SEO. They're willing to spend money and willing to create a lot of content. Does that equate to certainty of the best diagnostic expertise, treatment, patient care, and customer service? Sometimes. Sometimes not.

So, first, the best thing to do is make certain you get all your questions answered by the orthodontist and the practice's treatment coordinator. Don't hold back. Put them on the spot. Be assertive. Don't feel you have to be deferential to the doctor! Our goal in this is to have every patient and every patient's parent fully knowledgeable about every aspect of the treatment so that they have zero anxiety.

Now that we know where to get your most burning orthodontic questions answered, here are some simple tips we've amassed over the years to help you easily and effectively get the information you need:

How to Get Your Questions Answered

Make a list. The easiest way to get what you want is to know it in advance. Make a list of the various questions you have when they arise so you can quickly and easily go down the list to assure you've got the right answers for the right questions.

Bring it with you. Take the list with you when you go for your child's orthodontist visit. This way you have the questions at hand at the right place at the right time. If you're calling in to get answers, you can also have the list ready and tick off one question for every answer you receive.

Record the answers. If your orthodontist, or their receptionist, speaks too fast or you can't keep up while writing the answers down, why not record them? Your cell phone likely has a "record" feature and, if not, there are many affordable micro-recorders on the market today. This also allows you to replay the information for a decision maker that was not able to attend the exam.

Double-check. Finally, make sure you have the right answer by double-checking with your orthodontist or their team.

Knowing where to find the information you need is only half the battle; follow these tips and you'll know how to get what you're looking for as well.

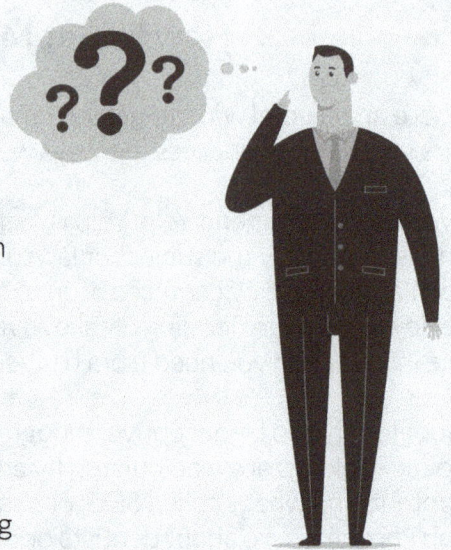

Regardless of how many questions you have, or your comfort level with technology, phone calls or in-person visits, your orthodontist should offer an option that fits your schedule and makes all your unresolved issues crystal clear.

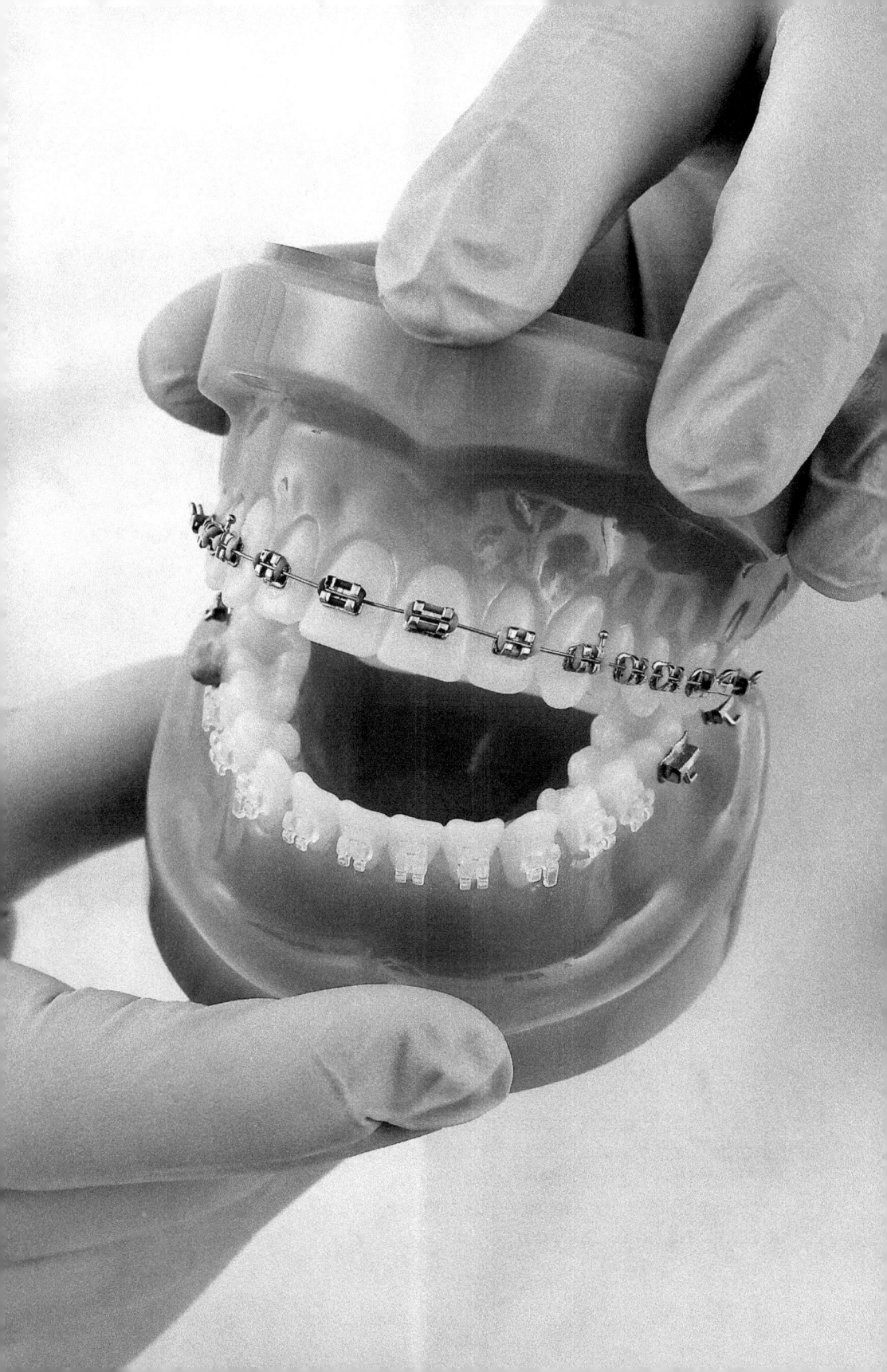

CHAPTER 7

How to Pay for Orthodontic Treatment and Braces

You may have never needed braces. You may have needed them and gotten them. Or you may be among the tens of thousands of people in our generation who needed them but did not get them, perhaps because your family decided they couldn't afford them. Maybe they didn't consider it a priority and probably underestimated the lifelong results of the decision. You may not only have lived with a "hide your smile" habit unnecessarily, but you may have developed chronic jaw pain and headaches, difficulty chewing, or even gum/periodontal disease that could have been prevented.

Regardless of which group you're in—and we hope it's not the third—we know you want to make the best choices for your son or daughter today, without being constrained just by the finances. Truth is, parents pay out the same cost for a number of different things not nearly as vital as health or emotional well-being without blinking, mostly because it's paid in installments or just never really *considered*, like the monthly cost for minutes/data on mobile devices, added up for a year or two. Now, compare this to the cost of braces and the total difference may not be that big. But, seeing the whole cost of orthodontic treatment all in one number may tempt thoughts of "maybe later" or "is this really necessary?"

We hope in the prior chapters we have succeeded at getting the "is it really necessary?" question erased. If there is visible need or if the orthodontist recommends treatment, it is necessary! It won't fix itself. It will probably get worse. It can negatively impact a person's health, emotional well-being, social life, and career. It can link to very serious medical problems. *Necessary* is not really debatable.

Now let's tackle the ugly matter of the money.

We say "ugly" because nobody really likes talking about this. Most orthodontists are nervous about it. Parents are uncomfortable with it. If there is a financial obstacle to treatment, most people are reluctant to admit it, offer other excuses, and then can't be helped by the doctor. We have to trust each other. With us, this discussion is entirely confidential, in a "safe zone." Orthodontists are not Martians, by the way; we have kids, college tuitions that loom, and family budgets.

What Is a Reasonable Fee and Cost?

A complete treatment program, including braces, can cost anywhere from $ 2,000 to $10,000 or so if it involves two phases. Most fall in between. Adjusted for inflation, these prices are actually **less than braces** decades ago, while the technology and quality has advanced. If you look at costs that could be avoided later, it makes sense to spend some now to prevent other problems from occurring.

For this investment, you will be getting the carefully selected, personalized solution to your child's irregularities and problems, prescribed using state-of-the-art digital technology along with the expertise of a specialist, and considerate, compassionate care from start to finish. Your investment includes a varying number of personalized appointments plus the orthodontic appliance itself and retainer care.

While it's never easy to part with such a sum, people do it every day for all sorts of less important things. Often, when they do pay for something like their new designer handbag, golf vacation, or suite of living room furniture, they'll pay for it outright or with their favorite credit card (getting the reward points in the bargain). If you put the orthodontic treatment program including braces on a typical credit card at the interest in play as we write this, and you choose to make only the minimum required monthly payment, your monthly payments will be relatively small. Even tight budgets can accommodate this when it is really important. It's less than most families pay for their cable and streaming entertainment. For many, if they got all their Starbucks stops consolidated into one monthly bill, it would be more than this!

Health Spending Accounts (HSA) /
Flex Spending Accounts (FSA)

The HSA allows you to set aside pre-tax dollars to be used for certain medical and health expenses for you or your family. If you have accumulated money in an HSA, you can probably spend it on orthodontic treatment. If you don't have an HSA, you might want to start one. Information can be found online about existing or new accounts and their rules of use, at www.healthcare.gov.

Other kinds of FSAs are typically set up through your place of employment and similarly enable you to set aside pre-tax dollars for medical expenses.

Sometimes, employers match contributions. Again, you can almost certainly tap funds from your FSA for your child's orthodontic care. Check with your employer about this.

If you have a tax accountant, you may want to consult with him about your HSA or FSA.

TIP: How can you make the most out of your employer's flex-pay plan?

First, make sure you understand how it works. Second, set aside flex-spending dollars in advance of need, and if possible, make the maximum contributions. Many employers allow higher limits than you'd think without asking, as much as $2,500 to $5,000 per year. Be aware of "family status changes" allowed by your plan that may enable you to change the amount being moved pre-tax from your paychecks to your account anytime during the year rather than just once at the first of the year—so you could bump up the amount in months before the first orthodontic treatment. IMPORTANT: Be aware of the balance and the loss of unused funds. In most cases, if you do not use these funds, you lose them, year to year. You usually have three months after the end of the calendar year to submit claims for eligible expenses from the previous year.

Insurance

These days, there are as many different types of insurance plans as there are patients in our office. We can't possibly speak to your unique and personal insurance policy without seeing it first but, in general, our experience tells us that "most" insurance policies cover "some" of your orthodontic expenses. We realize that answer sounds very vague, but here are a couple of variables you need to answer before an insurance agent can help you determine what, how long, and how many procedures fall under your insurance:

- The type of procedure (braces, Invisalign, etc.)

- The duration of the procedure (two months, six months, a year, etc.)

- The cause of the procedure (a patient presenting with pain, a parent's concern, traumatic injury or accident, congenital birth defect like cleft lip or palate etc.)

- The nature of the procedure (to correct pain/discomfort, cosmetic, etc.) We can only partially answer this question, but talking to your insurance agent will help you get the right answers you need.

TIP: Keep an insurance journal of every interaction with your carrier.

Write down the date, time of call, name of the person you contacted, and the exact instructions or recommendations following the call. Later, if your insurance company doesn't remember what they told you, you'll have it accurately written down. If they still don't remember, ask them to pull the recorded audio tape from your previous call, so that you can accurately "remind" them of exactly what they told you.

Loans

If you qualify, we offer Care Credit, which can provide an unsecured, signature-only loan for the treatment program, with repayment over twelve to sixty months. You don't need to go anywhere else to apply or do paperwork; we can take care of it in our office.

If you have equity in your home, the lowest-cost loan option may be a home equity line of credit or second mortgage. See your own bank, or check out RocketMortgage at rocket.quickenloans.com. As of this writing, mortgage interest is at record lows.

Obviously, a private loan from a family member can be the easiest option. A lot of preteens' and teens' important orthodontic care is financed at the Bank of Grandma and Grandpa.

If the other options are difficult or unavailable, we will set up a weekly, bimonthly, or monthly "paycheck payment plan" with a comfortable monthly payment.

What If You Really, Really Can't Afford Braces?

We have compiled a list of seventeen ways you may be able to substantially reduce the cost of braces. Frankly, some of them are less than ideal, and most are not available through our office, but they could be helpful if your back is really up against a financial wall.

1. **Get braces in April or November and see if you can save a little extra by paying in full.** These are the months that orthodontists are the least-busy, and it's when we have our most meetings (April–

May). In November, everyone is getting ready for the holidays or the office is closed the week of Thanksgiving. By scheduling during the "off season," you can often find better deals with willing orthodontists.

2. **See if you can get a discount for not breaking any brackets.** Believe it or not, most orthodontists would happily take $100 off your final bill if you don't break any appliances throughout treatment!

3. **New technology; better pricing.** See if you can be one of your orthodontist's first patients with a new technology and save some money on the lab fee or receive a discount for being a teaching case.

4. **Ask your insurance plans when they send out their fee schedules to participating providers.** If the insurance company updates their fees or the orthodontist raises his or her fees to keep up with the cost of inflation, it might be around November in preparation for the next year.

5. **See your dentist every four to six months.** While you're wearing your braces, the extra cleaning each year can prevent tooth decay, a costly item to repair.

6. **Get your flex spending dollars in order with your employer.** If you set money aside in a flex plan, it may be "tax-free" but it comes with some stipulations: namely, you have to use it before the end of the year or else you lose it.

7. **See if you can get a second set of retainers from your orthodontist at the end of treatment.** Sometimes getting two sets of retainers at the same time can be cheaper than buying a second set later in life when you lose or break your first set.

8. **See if your husband or wife has an insurance plan that covers braces.** Be sure to enroll in the plan with enough time to spare before your child needs braces, so that the procedure is not denied by your insurance company due to a waiting period.

9. **Ask for flexible financing options.** When you boil it down to the basics, your orthodontist really just wants to help you. Regardless of his specialty, your doctor spent way too much time in school not to love what he does. If you're easy to work with, keep your teeth clean and avoid breaking your braces while you're wearing them, he or she

will probably be thrilled to help you finance the care, or find another way to afford the investment.

10. **Do you have multiple kids in treatment?** If so, take advantage of that fact and see if you can get a family discount.

11. **If finances are extremely tight, you should check out the organizations that orthodontists have created to help provide pro-bono care, such as SmilesChangeLives.org.** There are even more foundations like this if you have a cleft palate or other facial anomalies, like the Rheam Foundation for Cleft and Craniofacial Research.

12. **School auctions, churches, or public service entities will often receive donations from local orthodontists wishing to donate a case to the school or organization for a fundraiser.** Checking around local school newsletters or church bulletins for their upcoming silent auctions could be a great find! If you're unwilling to leave such things to chance, call your local schools or churches and ask them specifically if they have such a fund and, if so, how to apply/qualify.

13. **If you're thinking about a career change, apply at your local orthodontist's office.** Most orthodontists offer free or discounted braces to their team and their children as an employee benefit! (And you never know, you could love your career *and* your child's new braces!)

14. **Military, schoolteachers and firefighters sometimes receive special courtesies in dental and orthodontic offices throughout the year.** Keep your ears open and you might save a few bucks or at least get a donation from the orthodontist to your organization.

15. **This tactic won't save you any money, but it could earn your organization or business some money if you have a newsletter, sports team, fund-raiser, or special event that needs a sponsor.** Ask your orthodontist. Most orthodontic offices are huge supporters of the communities in which they practice and would probably love to advertise with your organization.

16. **Got taxes?** Good! Why not use your tax refund to help pay for treatment in full and ask for a courtesy on the average fees associated with financing a full orthodontic case? In some areas, you can save as

much as 10 percent on the cost of braces by simply saving your pennies and paying the entire bill at once, up front.

17. **Ask for more flexible financing, through a third-party credit company like Chase Healthcare Advance, through CareCredit, or by using in-house financing through your orthodontist.** Most orthodontists will accept a reasonable down payment and split the remaining amount into easy monthly payments for your convenience. With automated withdrawals from a checking or savings account, you might be able to stretch the monthly payments out over a longer period to make each payment lower. Just don't be shocked if your orthodontist asks you to approve a credit check. A little homework up front can be well worth the effort when your monthly orthodontic bill is lower than your cell phone bill!

There's no doubt about it; braces can be expensive. However, now that you're armed with these seventeen massive, budget-saving tips, you won't need to decide between braces and your budget ever again!

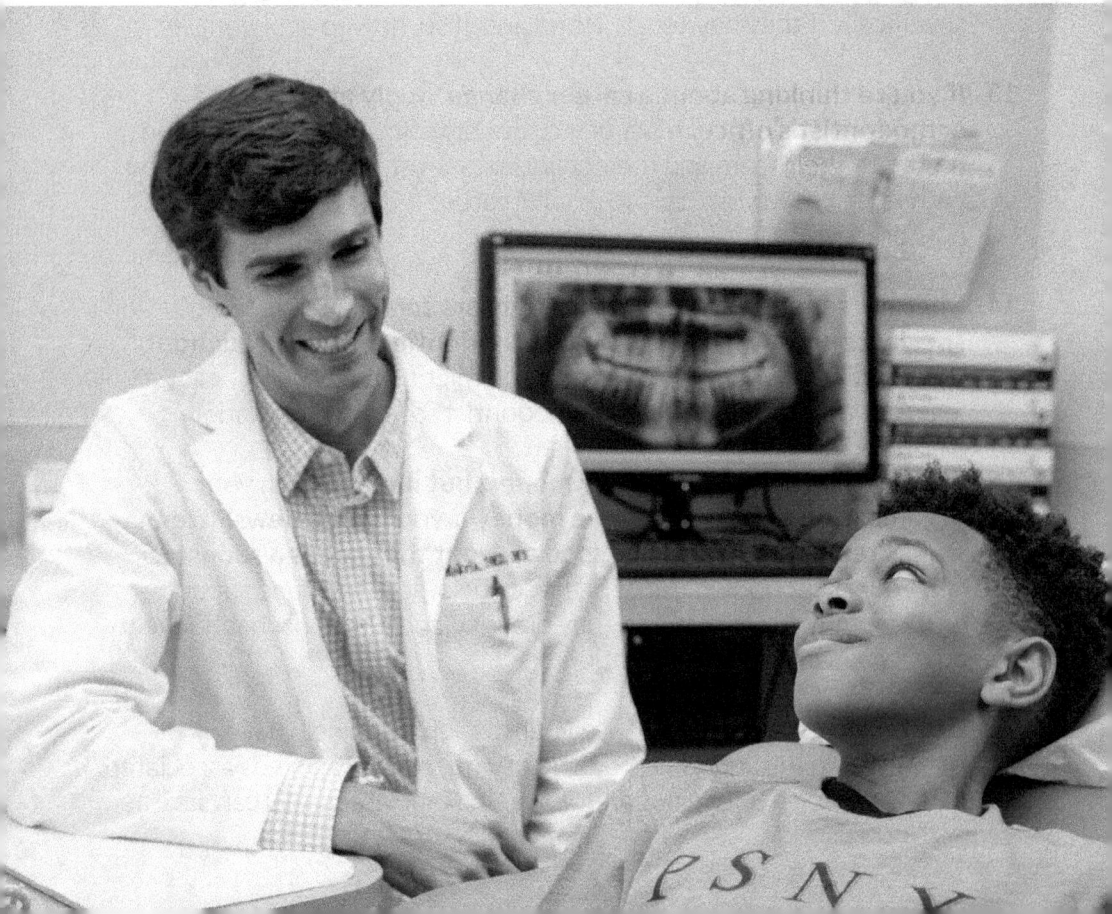

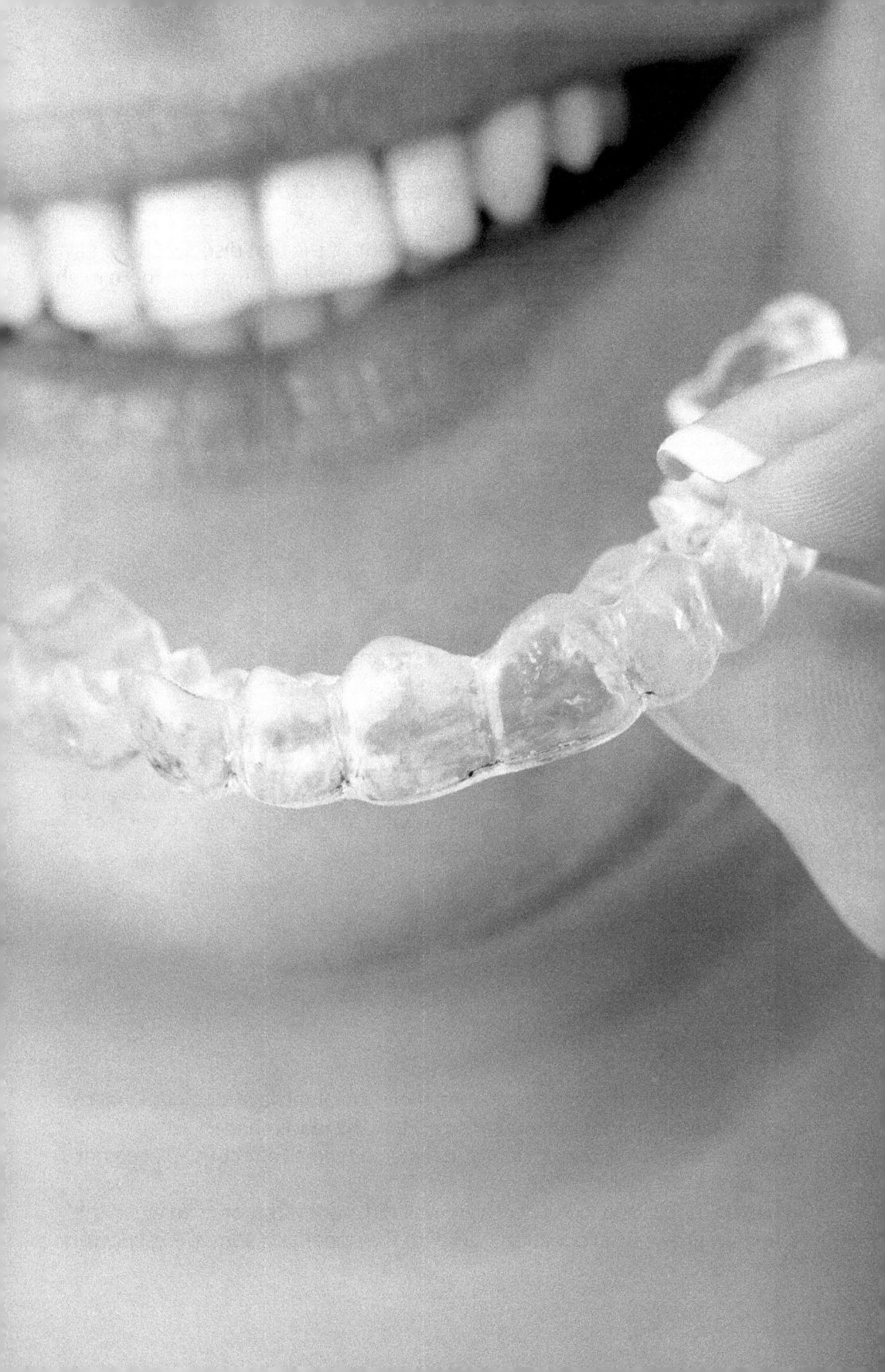

CHAPTER 8

What Are the Treatment Options?

If your child is ready for orthodontic care, one of the first discussions to have with your orthodontist is which procedure is right for him or her; there might be more options than you had ever imagined.

If you're like most people, you associate orthodontists with braces, but these days that is just one arm of what we or any orthodontist does. Here are some of the services most orthodontists will provide their patients with during the course of routine treatment:

- Metal braces
- Invisalign clear removable aligners
- Clear braces
- Expanders to match jaw size and tooth size
- Habit appliances to eliminate thumb sucking
- Space maintainers
- Retainers to prevent crowding and shifting of teeth
- Functional appliances to help improve facial balance
- Early treatment and growth modification
- Customized appliances designed uniquely for each patient

While many of these services may seem self-explanatory to you, several will probably not. In the following pages, we will try to elaborate on several of them, including:

- Crossbite correction
- Metal braces
- Clear braces
- Invisalign

Crossbite Correction

As your child's teeth begin to grow in, there's a lot more at work than mere gum lines, tooth fairies, and molar size. How the jaw is shaped, when it develops, and even how "normally" it develops can all affect the placement and comfort of your child's teeth.
When the upper and lower teeth grow at different rates, or even when the lower jaw grows disproportionately with the upper jaw, something known as a "crossbite" can occur.

> *Your child might have a crossbite if, for instance, the lower jaw is out of line with the upper jaw (kind of like a box that won't close right because one of the hinges is bent).*

Or maybe your child's upper and lower jaws are out of alignment so instead of the top and bottom front teeth meeting "naturally" as they should, the front teeth fall somewhat behind the lower teeth. This would be an underbite or the reverse of an overbite.

As you might imagine, any or all of these developments can lead to short- and long-term discomfort for your child.

How, When, and Why Crossbites Form

You might be amazed to find out how many ways a crossbite can form as your child grows and develops during his or her formative years. Heredity is one key to jaw growth, or alignment, as is the size of your child's developing jaw.

Another factor that can contribute to the development of a potential crossbite is if it takes your child too long to lose his or her baby teeth. In some extreme cases, if it takes too long for your child to lose his baby teeth, another set of teeth can grow in behind them, throwing the alignment off and contributing to a crossbite.

Believe it or not, something as basic as whether your child breathes through her nose or her mouth can also contribute to a crossbite. While most children breathe through their noses, some children develop a habit early on of breathing through their mouths instead.

In children who breathe through their noses while they're sleeping, the tongue naturally rests on the roof of the mouth, promoting natural and proper upper jaw growth. When young children breathe through their mouths, however, the tongue relocates from the roof of the mouth to the bottom, removing that extra support and potentially contributing to reduced upper jaw bone growth; this can create the crossbite we spoke of previously.

Thumb Habit

There is a high correlation with thumb-sucking and crossbites. The resulting force of the cheeks on the upper back teeth as the thumb is sucked causes a "narrowing" of the upper dental arch. This can result in a crossbite.

How Can I Spot a Crossbite?

Although it sounds severe and even painful from the description provided earlier, the effects of a crossbite can take time to manifest themselves. Still, here are some of the telltale signs your child might be cultivating, or already suffering from, a crossbite:

- Snoring
- Difficulty breathing
- Chewing on one side of the mouth or the other
- Bottom teeth are in front on top teeth when biting down
- If your child's chin seems "off center" or disproportionate

How, When, and Why to Correct a Crossbite

Where should you start looking for treatment if you're concerned about your child's jaw development after reading this section? If you suspect your child might have a crossbite, call an orthodontist for a consultation.

There are many possible treatments available for a crossbite, and your orthodontist can work with you closely to make the right and specific decisions for you and your child.

When should you have it evaluated? You know our standard answer when it comes to questions like this one: as early as possible! The same way a fire fighter would tell you to take care of a faulty microwave, electrical wiring or space heater sooner rather than later, we will most often favor early treatment to later.

Crossbites are often closely linked with other orthodontic issues, such as teeth alignment, jaw size, and growth, so naturally, the sooner you address any or all of these issues, the better.

Finally, why should you address a crossbite? Crossbites can lead to pain, discomfort, asymmetric growth, and a lack of confidence as your child begins to feel insecure because of this very treatable problem.

Not only can crossbites become physically uncomfortable if left untreated, but if the misalignment or root cause of the bite isn't fixed early in childhood, then the child's appearance and, ultimately, confidence could be affected as the crossbite becomes more pronounced in adolescence.

"Our son has a lot of anxiety about visiting any doctor, but the transition into the orthodontics world was very easy and painless for our family. Thank you for all that you do to bring beautiful smiles to our family and many, many more!" — Molly H.

Metal Braces

The fact is, metal braces still have a valued place in the orthodontic world, and despite advances and breakthroughs of products like Invisalign and even clear braces, they aren't going extinct anytime soon! This is because metal braces are very strong and can withstand most types of treatment. Today's metal braces are smaller, sleeker, and more polished than ever before.

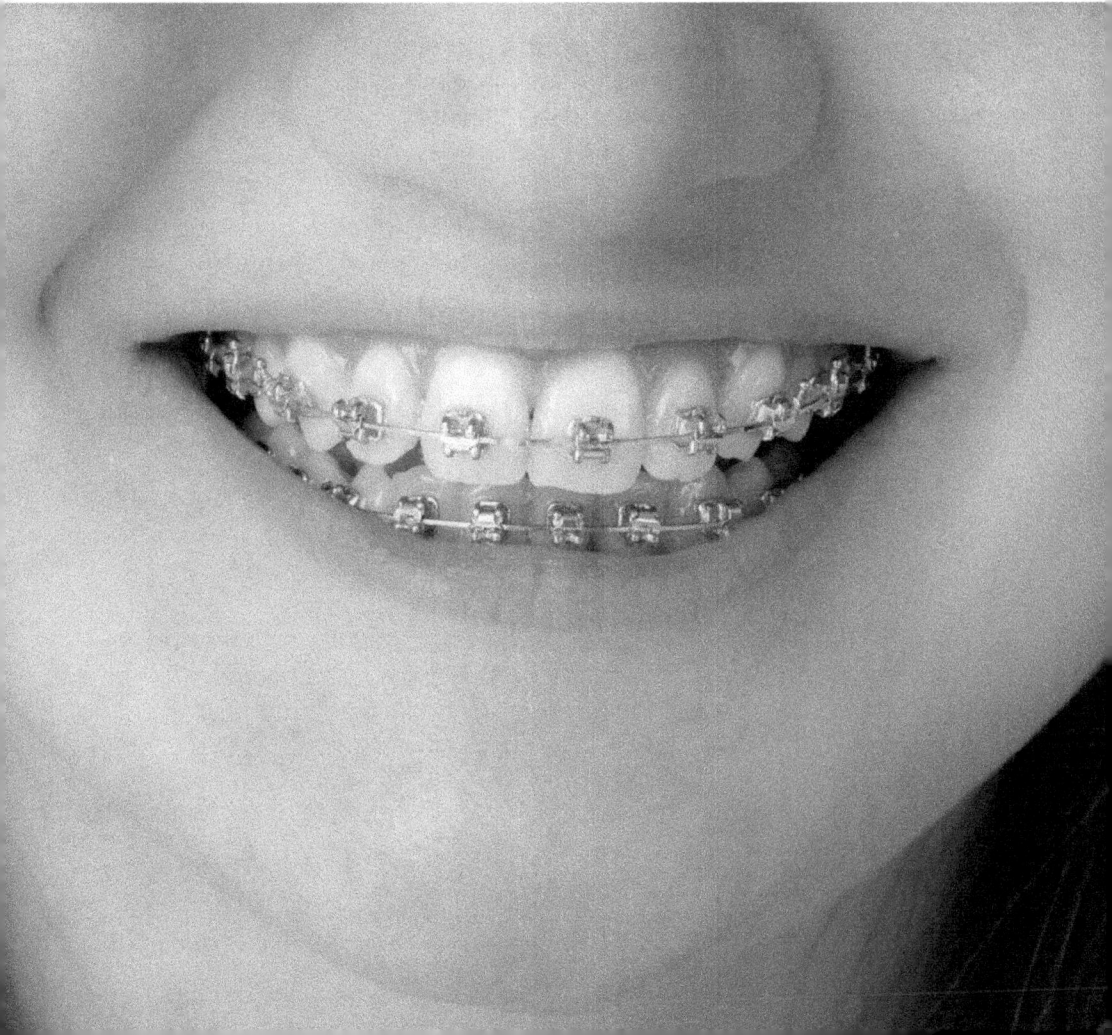

Clear Braces

Ceramic braces are very strong and generally do not stain. Some adults like to choose ceramic braces because they "blend in" with the teeth and are less noticeable than metal. These are the type of braces that actor Tom Cruise had.

Adult Orthodontics

It's not uncommon for individuals who have undergone orthodontic treatment earlier in life to find their teeth have drifted out of alignment over the years. Most adults won't think twice about bleaching their teeth to roll back the effects of time. Yet few think about the role orthodontics can play.

Adults of all ages can enjoy the same cosmetic and health benefits of properly aligned teeth.

Improperly aligned teeth can do more than undermine your confidence. They can make proper cleaning and brushing more difficult, contribute to enamel loss and even set the stage for more significant problems down the road.

The Solution Is Clear

Orthodontists believe every individual has the right to live their life with a smile they truly love. Healthy, straight, and attractive smiles can make you or your child happier and more self-confident. And isn't that what we all want?

Embrace the confidence that comes with beautifully aligned teeth and put your smile on display. Schedule a consultation to see which treatment option is right for you.

Invisalign

Invisalign is a widely advertised, well-known, and popular orthodontic product, and often, kids know about it and ask parents and doctors for it by name. For many, it's as good an option as any other and sometimes even the best option.

Invisalign uses advanced, proprietary 3-D computer imaging technology to "map" the entire span of treatment, from the present teeth alignment to the desired positioning, alignment, and smile. Clear aligners are custom made and based on the 3-D imaging. Invisalign has many features that have helped make it such a popular choice. The aligners are removable, even before a snack or meal as well as for general hygiene. There are no metal brackets or wires. Office visits for adjustments throughout the treatment program are fast, easy and painless. The thermoplastic aligners are virtually invisible. Over one million patients have been treated with Invisalign, and there is a special Invisalign system for teens.

Because Invisalign is computer mapped, there's sometimes the idea that anybody can install Invisalign and that all practitioners using Invisalign are the same. I have an important warning about this: during each stage of the complete treatment, only certain teeth are allowed to move. Which teeth move in what order, and the amount of time (days/weeks) needed for each successive set of aligners differs for each patient. This is why you rely on an expert orthodontist. At the start, we determine whether you or your son or daughter would be a good candidate for the Invisalign approach, or if you would be better served with a different appliance. You have to rely on somebody to tell you. I promise you, there are kids who've been hurried to Invisalign who were not good candidates for it.

Invisalign Teen

Much like the standard adult version, the Invisalign Teen system lets you do it the modern, hygienic way. Your new smile is created with the most innovative technology—a series of clear aligners that are custom-fit to your teeth.

The first thing you should know is that your treatment can begin even if you don't have all of your permanent teeth. Invisalign Teen was designed to meet your needs.

Invisalign Teen aligners will snap on your child's teeth easily. They are comfortable and practically invisible. Invisalign Teen allows for permanent teeth to grow in gently and it continuously moves teeth in small increments. Aligners are worn for about two weeks and then swapped for a new pair.

Invisalign Teen aligners have a "Blue Dot Wear Indicator," designed to show an estimation of wear time. The dot is designed to fade until it's clear over a two-week period if you wear your aligners properly (meaning for twenty to twenty-two hours every day).

Invisalign Teen is designed to custom-fit to your child's teeth and go with his or her lifestyle. During treatment, your child can keep smiling, playing sports, eating what he or she wants, and brushing and flossing normally. Plus, unlike traditional braces, the aligners are made of smooth plastic and move teeth gradually.

The aligners can be removed for eating, brushing, and flossing or going to a special event. The aligners are replaceable if lost. That's right; you get up to six free individual aligners.

After your child's Invisalign Teen treatment, you may find his or her self-confidence boosted by their new smile and the change in their appearance. Some people even feel that way during the treatment. As you know, smiling has many benefits. It can help your child make a strong impression in lots of different social situations—at school, at work, or at a party.

Invisalign Teen really works. It helps correct a broad range of dental and orthodontic issues. You can get a confident smile without metal brackets or wires. It works on many kinds of conditions, including overly crowded or widely spaced teeth, crossbites, overbites, and underbites.

We've used Invisalign to successfully transform the smiles of many patients, but we do not prescribe it to everybody. After all, popularity should not govern medical care!

Trustworthy, Objective Advice

Coastline Orthodontics is not obligated to any providers of different braces products and technologies. We select and recommend what we believe is the most appropriate and beneficial choice for your child. We are happy to discuss the pros and cons of different choices, if your child has his/her heart set on, say, Invisalign, because that's what a friend has, or based on information you've obtained.

Call us at 904.600.4749 or go to www.coastlineorthodontics.com to schedule your own Customized Smile Analysis.

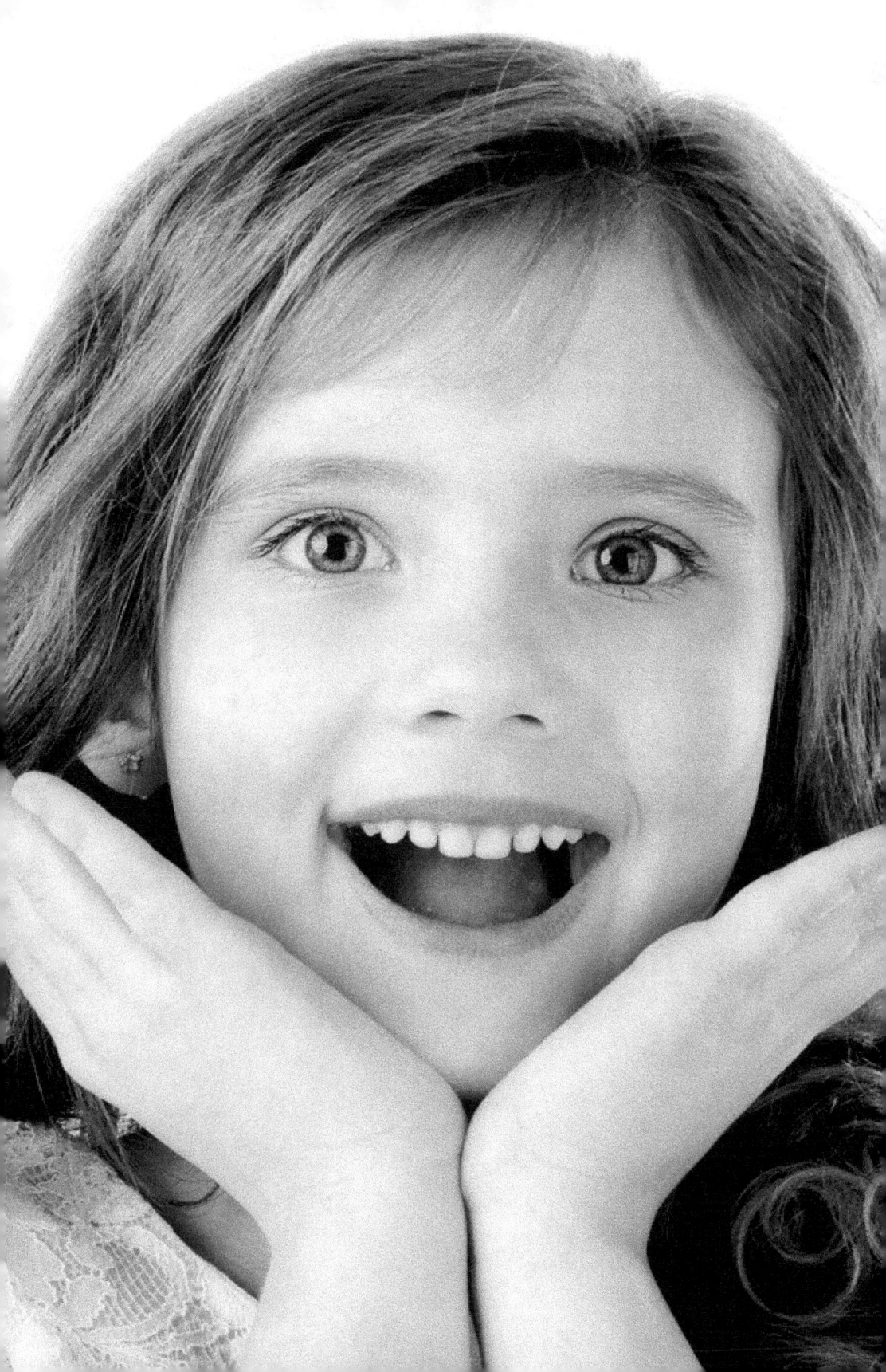

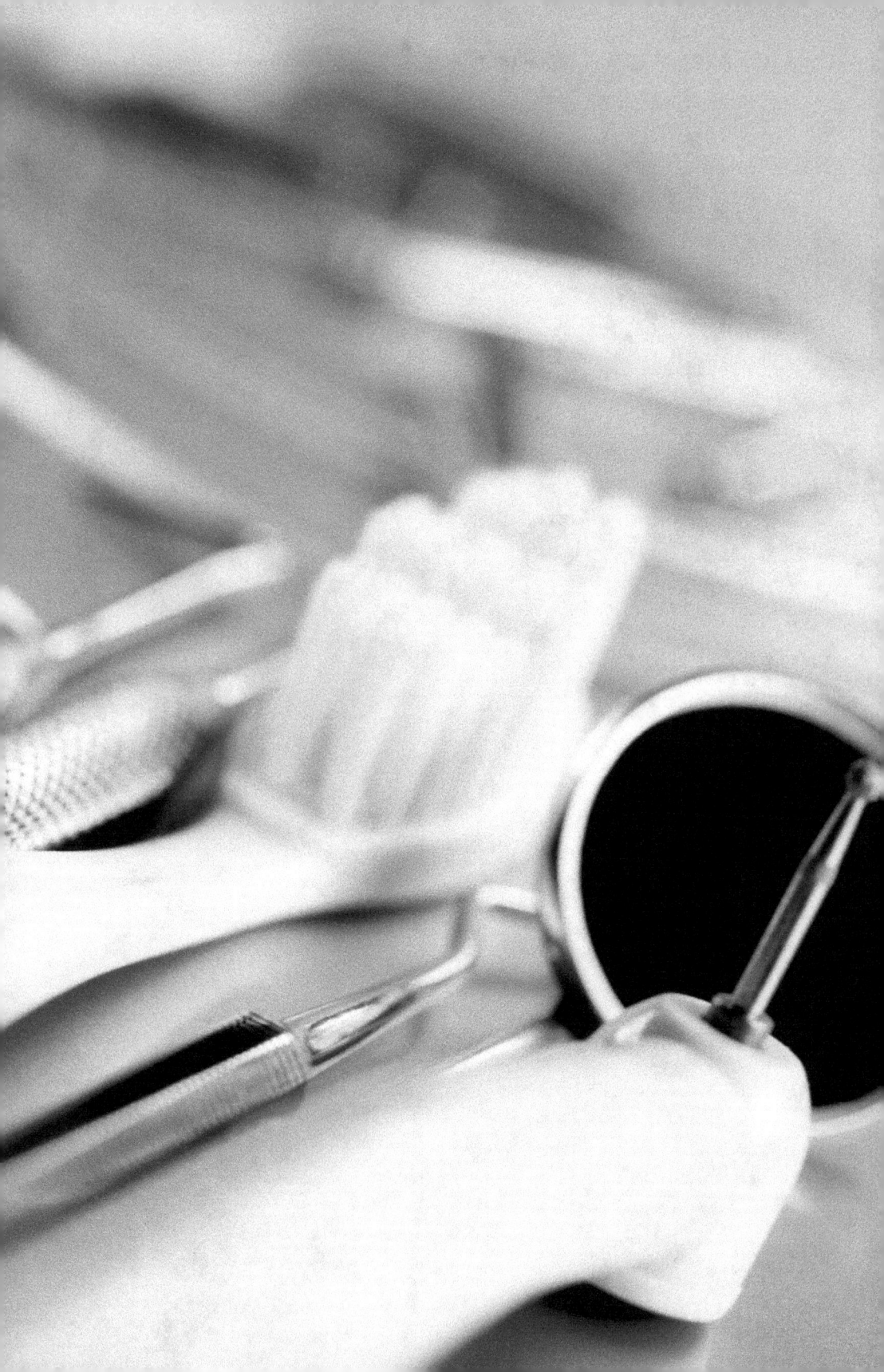

CHAPTER 9

How Difficult Is Living With Braces?

Remember, this *isn't* 1982. Or 1992. Today's braces aren't anything like yours if you had them decades ago. Today's orthodontic care is far more advanced, more sophisticated, and more patient-centered than any prior generation has experienced. If you had traditional metal braces twenty years or so ago, you experienced medieval torture. The dungeon is gone too, replaced by ultra-modern, comfortable offices. Out of the dark, into the light!

Living with a child in braces is not going to be anywhere near as difficult as you might imagine.

Let's look at a few specific concerns.

Brushing and Hygiene

Modern braces, whether they're metal, flexible, or "invisible," are all actually made to fit the individual and facilitate easy, painless, thorough brushing. This means your child brushes pretty much the same as he would if he didn't have braces.

Here are some simple tips you can share with your child for the best results when brushing with braces on:

- Brush your teeth in the morning, after you eat and before bed*
- Brush, rinse, and look; if you find any areas that are not clean, brush them again.
- Brush your gums as you brush your teeth (massage and stimulate).
- Take extra care in the area between the gums and the braces, because food caught and left there can cause swollen gums, cavities, discomfort, and permanent teeth stains.
- If no toothpaste is available, brush without.
- If you are unable to brush, rinse your mouth vigorously with water.
- Replace your old toothbrush when it gets worn out.
- It's absolutely essential you continue regular visits to your family dentist for checkups and cleanings throughout your orthodontic treatment!

* At our office, you'll be provided with a home kit including an electric toothbrush, toothpaste, and rinse.

Depending on the age of your child, you, the parent, may need to supervise the first few brushings with the braces in place. You should not have a whining, resistant, difficult child on your hands because of any of this. It should be painless, simple, and routine.

Forbidden Foods Your Child Must Avoid

After your child's orthodontic appliance/braces have been placed, the teeth are usually "tender" and sensitive for as few as three to as many as ten days: a *short* time. During these few days, softer foods are recommended: soups, macaroni, spaghetti, eggs, fish, Jell-O, yogurt. As needed, Tylenol or Advil are adequate in relieving any discomfort.* Warm saltwater rinses can be helpful. We also provide a "soft white wax," a safe topical that eases soft tissue discomfort.

For the entire duration of the braces being in place, I'd advise your child to stay away from hard and sticky foods that can damage braces and may lengthen the time they have to be worn or even require extra office visits. Sugar-rich foods can make hygiene harder and cause calculus build-up and cavities. You're probably already monitoring and limiting your child's intake of such foods, so there's really nothing new under the sun here. But, for the record, here are the "featured items" that should be avoided during orthodontic treatment and wearing of braces:

1. **Rock-hard foods:** Ice (don't chew ice!), nuts, popcorn (has hard kernels inside), peanut brittle, rock candy, whole apples and carrots (unless cut into bite sized pieces), corn on the cob, hard pretzels, hard rolls, hard taco shells.

2. **Extra-sticky foods:** Jolly Ranchers or Starbursts or similar candies, bubble gum, taffy, and sticky Cinnabon rolls.

3. **Very chewy foods:** Pizza crust, beef jerky, gummy bears.

---

* Prescription pain pills with dangerous side effects are not needed. Any orthodontist or dentist easily prescribing such drugs is not to be trusted. As you are no doubt aware from the news, opioid addiction is rampant. Pain drugs are, contrary to early assertions by their manufacturers, proving to be extremely addictive, for many people after nominal and legitimate use.

Note: No chewing on pencils or pens.

4. **Super-sugary foods and drinks should be limited:** Soda with sugar, ice cream, most cookies and cake. Yes, these can be the worst of the forbidden foods if consumed frequently. Some kids will give you a tough time. But there are sugar-free versions of all these kinds of foods, to be made or baked, or store-bought.

We will speak about this with your son or daughter and give them a printed list, but you will have to reinforce, monitor, and provide some substitute foods to prevent mutiny or months of sulking. Most kids get it, though, when they understand these foods are linked to their treatment outcome and the length of time they are in treatment. Most parents who are initially really worried about this tell us later it wasn't the horror show they'd imagined.

Emergencies, Injuries, Travel, and Time Away from Home

Many "emergencies" actually aren't and can be easily and safely remedied at home. You are provided with information on what to do in case of an emergency, and you can always access the same information at our web site, 24/7/365.

If you do run up against an emergency that isn't easily managed with these instructions or can't wait for regular office hours, we have a special phone number to call that routes to a knowledgeable staff member directly or with a quick return call.

If your family or son or daughter are away from home and say, they chomp down on a piece of toffee and break a piece of their braces, there is always a remedy. You are not going to cut your vacation short and rush to the airport! Again, often a remedy you do by our instructions can meet the urgent need until everybody gets back home.

Sports

Speaking of injuries, the question of sports versus braces worries kids and parents alike. These days, kids are very active in organized and school sports, some starting one as another's season is ending. You know this; you are coordinating the schedules and working as their unpaid chauffeur.

Good news: for every sport and every level of play, there is either an inexpensive off-the-shelf mouth guard or a slightly costlier, custom-fit mouth guard to provide an extra, suitable level of dental protection and to protect the braces themselves. In some sports, additional face masks or other equipment normally treated as an option can be added and used during the time period of the orthodontic treatment. Ask us for guidance for your child and their sport(s). Some mouth guards even come with insurance against dental injury, covering financial costs.

By the way, there are collegiate and pro athletes, even NFL players, getting orthodontic treatment and even wearing braces. If they can, your child can! You do not need the drama of stopping your child from playing the sports they're committed to because of their orthodontic treatment.

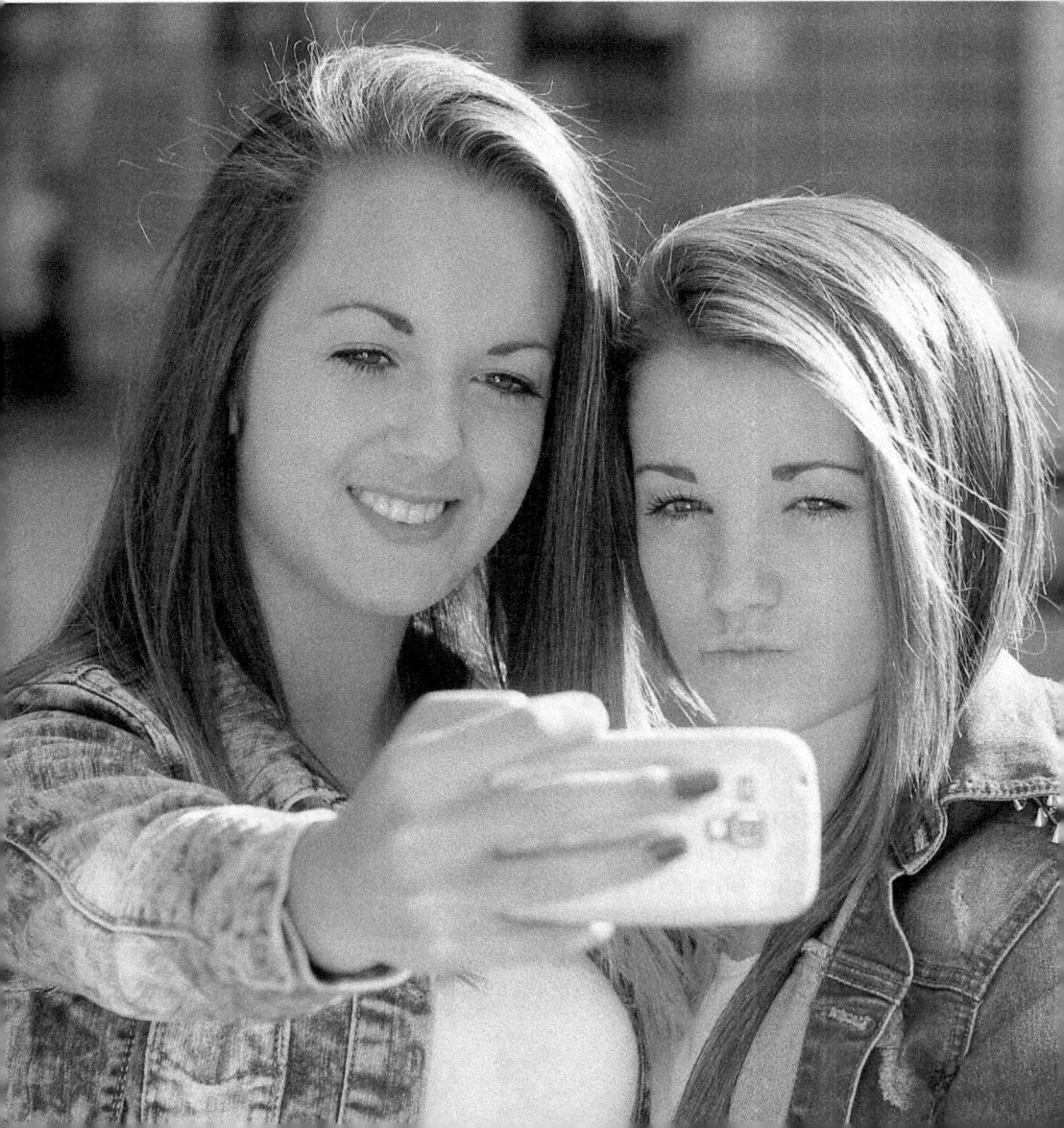

Tips for Helping Your Child Adjust to a Life with Braces

- **All the cool kids are doing it (or soon will be):** Braces are a very popular appliance during the middle school and high school years.

  Rather than focus on how he or she feels wearing braces, encourage your child to begin actively looking for other kids who are wearing braces. Chances are, they'll find lots more than they ever imagined!

- **Even famous people do it:** Gwen Stefani. Prince Harry. Drew Barrymore. Tom Cruise. Dakota Fanning. Danny Glover. The list of famous people who've worn braces—many of them as adults—could fill half this book. Share with your child how even the most famous people in the spotlight sometimes need a little help through braces.

- **Fast forward:** Have your child focus on the "after" when he or she gets down about the "before" shots!

- **Be prepared:** Finally, create a "master list" of things your child likes to do: things that make him feel special, confident, brave, calm, relaxed, or excited. If you notice him feeling down, consult your list and make plans to do something special in the near future to boost his confidence level back to where you know it belongs!

Call us at 904.600.4749 or go to www.coastlineorthodontics.com to schedule your own Customized Smile Analysis.

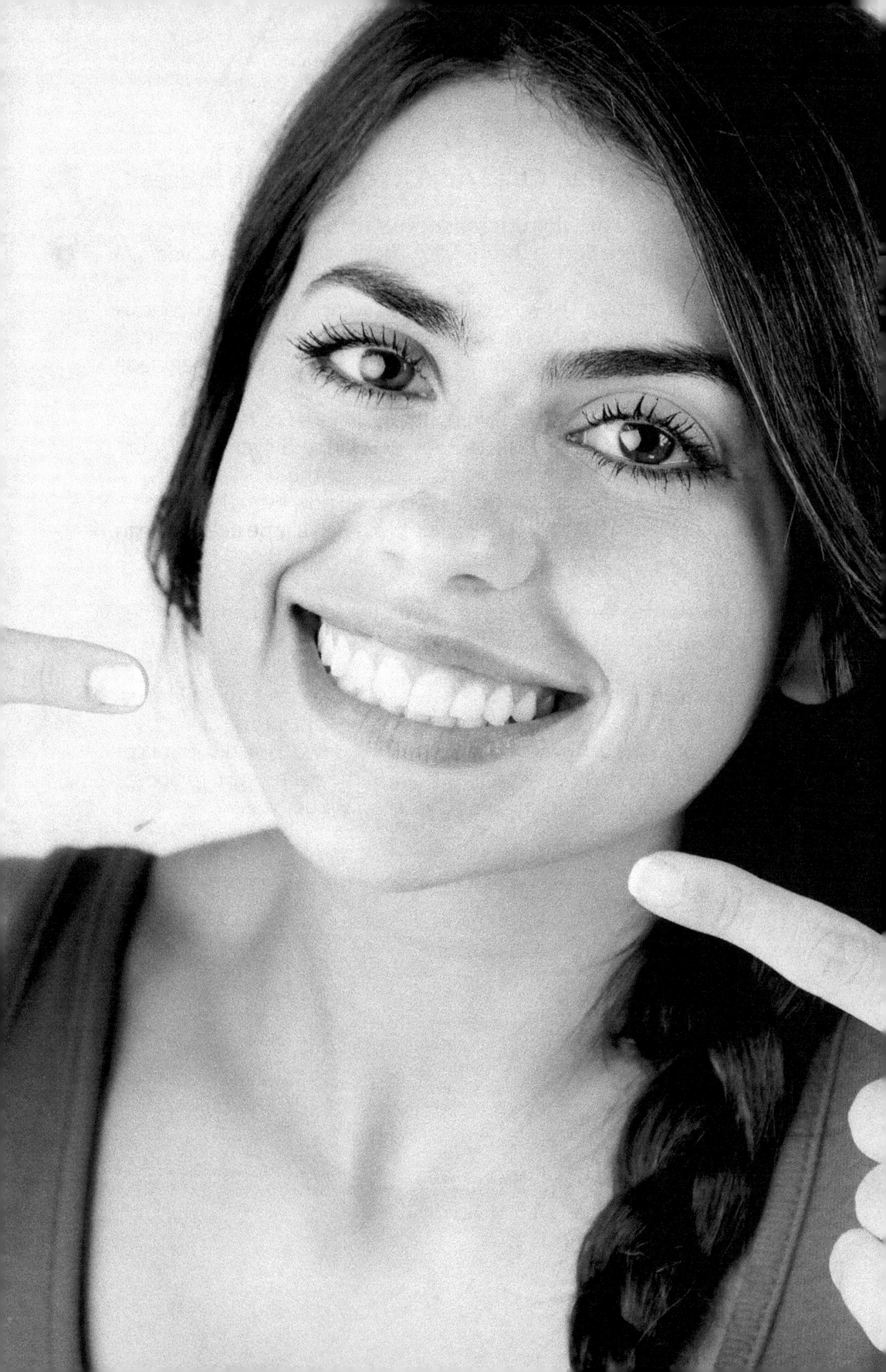

CHAPTER 10

Life After Braces: Retainers

So, your child's braces are off and they're ready to live a life full of confidence and good oral health. They may think, I'm free! I'm free! Well, not quite yet. The selection of the right braces, the expert orthodontist, and the compliant wearing of the braces gets us about three-fourths of the way to where we want to be: a well-aligned, as-perfect-as-possible, healthy smile for life. But after braces, there are retainers.

While many patients are understandably eager to be done with braces once they come off, the fact is, retainers do as much work—if not more—than the braces themselves. Straight teeth in proper alignment have to stay that way, and for that, retainers are a big help.

When the braces are removed, teeth can still shift if not helped through a period of adjustment, to settle in. Retainers gently but purposefully remind the teeth to stay straight during this adjustment period. It's advised that nearly all patients who've gone through the time, work, and expense of braces will want to use fixed or removable retainers for months or years or even for life and continue to schedule regular orthodontic check-ups. Some dentists doing braces won't tell you this, but we will. Years ago, clinicians believed that once teeth were straightened by braces, they would simply stay that way forever. New science says otherwise. In fact, shifting of teeth as we age is to be expected. Teeth naturally shift to the middle and crowd. So, retainers are actually extremely important in maintaining the new smile from braces.

Any claims otherwise, by some "brand" of braces or any doctor, are flat-out false.

Retainers can play a role in:

- Closing any gaps that may remain in the bite

- Correcting any speech problems—sometimes occurring with a new bite or jaw position

- Tongue thrust—where the tongue slips under the teeth while talking

- Bruxism—grinding teeth while sleeping

As you can see, there's a lot more to this than just "installing and removing braces."

We tend to decide on the best kind of retainer for your child before the removal of the braces. Growth of the jaw following treatment (yes, the jaw is still growing in adolescents, to age eighteen or so), stabilization of the gums and bone tissues, pressures from lips and tongue, and other factors tell us what type of retainer should be worn and for how long. Retainers are made out of plastic, and sometimes, still metal. They are custom made and fit, as part of the complete orthodontic treatment. However, after the initial orthodontic exam, at the same time the best braces are being selected, it's usually possible, with a good degree of certainty, to predict the type of retainer(s) your child is going to need, and we are happy to share that information with you at that time.

Some retainers are invisible or nearly invisible. These are clear plastic retainers. A fixed retainer is typically placed on the inside/back surfaces of the lower front teeth. A fixed retainer may be used until lower jaw growth is complete and then no longer needed. When your child hears "retainer" he will most likely picture a removable retainer. These make hygiene easy, are easily removed and cleaned daily and can be removed for a sports activity. There are even "fashion retainers" now—popular with kids of different ages— in school colors, and some even with pictures on them!

This is an important part of braces aftercare and part of the complete orthodontic treatment program personalized for your child.

Call us at 904.600.4749 or go to www.coastlineorthodontics.com to schedule your own Customized Smile Analysis.

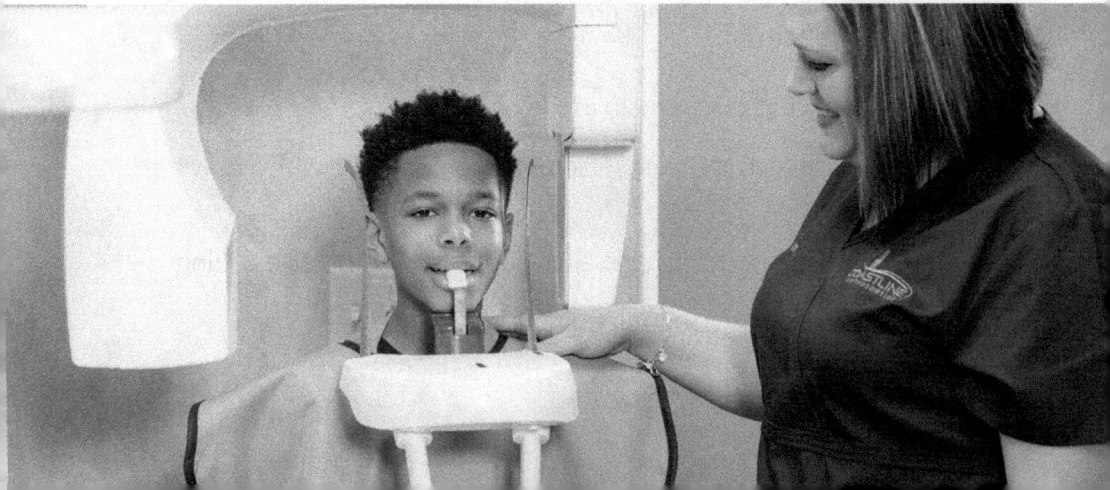

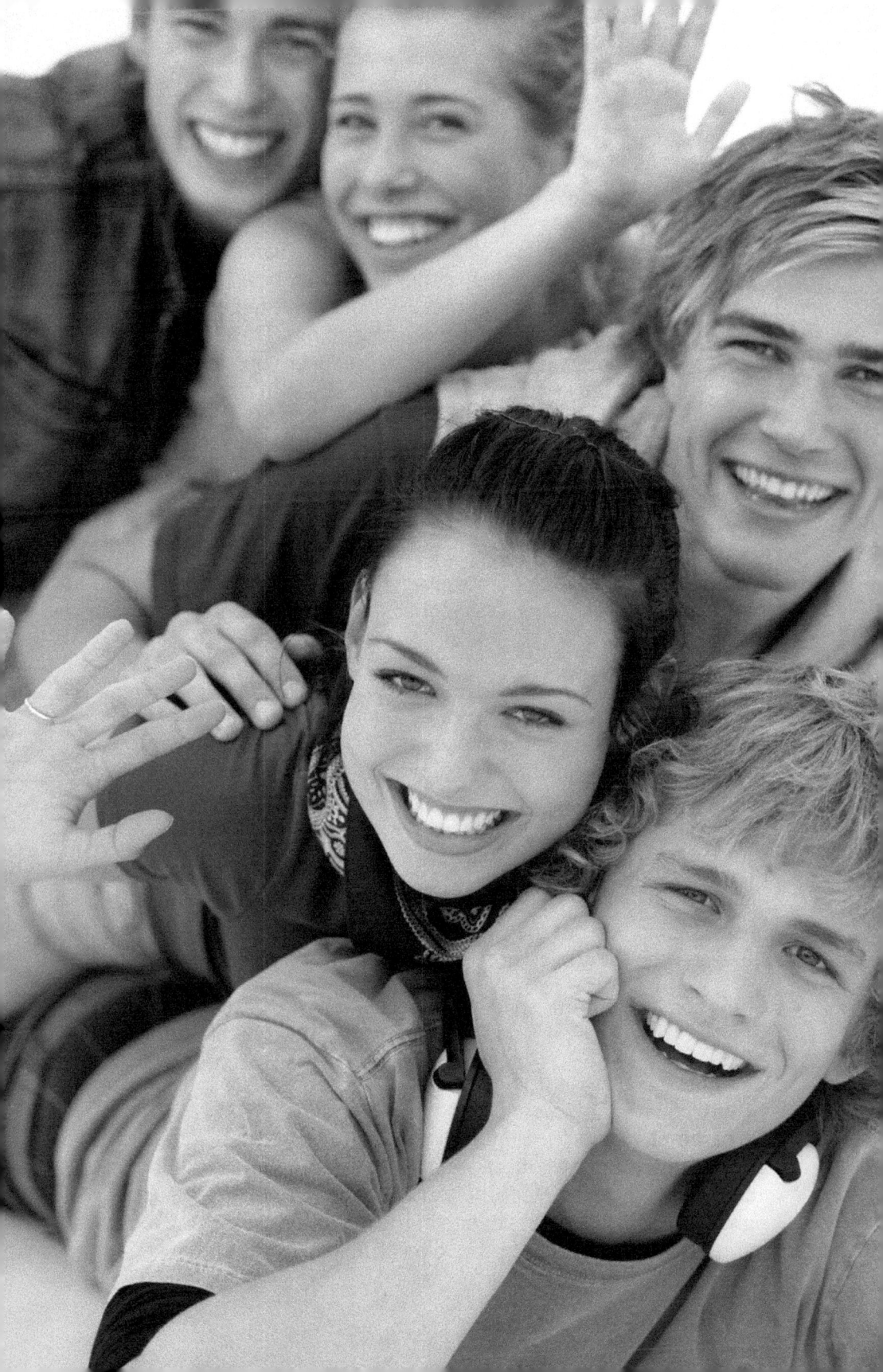

CHAPTER 11

Let's Celebrate!

Having to wear braces can last for six months to two years or more in certain cases. During the time your child has them, they may have moved from child to preteen or preteen to teen. At times, they may have felt embarrassed by having them, and possibly missed out on some things. They probably gave up favorite foods and snacks. They at least had to be super-conscious of what they ate and didn't eat. It's been a long time since they could sink their teeth into an apple!

You endured whatever complaining there was. You traded time to the office visits. You dealt with the "uh-oh!" and "now what did you do?" emergencies if there were any. And, of course, you paid the bill.

We like to see our patients celebrate getting their braces off. There are so many ways your child can celebrate, everything from writing a journal about their experience to recording a video that shares their experience and shows their new look.

Here are a few options your child may want to consider:

- **Throw a party.** Throwing a "braces are off" party is a great way to celebrate. They can invite their friends over, put out the foods that they've been longing for, and they can enjoy showing off those new straight teeth. Their friends will love being able to take part in the celebration.

- **Plan a photo shoot.** Your child deserves to show the world their new beautiful smile! Plan a photo shoot, so they can be one-on-one with a photographer and put their best smile forward. They'll get some great shots and can show all their friends on social media their new look.

- **Chew some gum.** Your child might have wanted to have gum for the longest time. Although it's not the best habit, they can take an afternoon to chew some gum and feel guilt and worry free. Chew to your heart's content!

- **Go caramel.** Now is the time your child can sink his teeth into something like a caramel apple. No more avoiding the caramel and cutting the apple into bite-sized pieces. Nope, he can actually eat a full caramel apple, right off the stick! He can get one at the mall or a carnival or even make them himself. Either way, he'll love being able to bite into that sticky gooey sweetness worry free!

- **Picnic.** A picnic in the park will make for a fun celebration. Take some of your child's favorite outdoor games, invite the friends, and have a cooler filled with icy drinks. On the grill, you can plan for things like corn on the cob that your child had to largely avoid while having braces. It will make for a memorable afternoon!

- **Have a potluck dinner.** Have your child's friends and family each bring a dish that could not have been enjoyed with braces. This will give them the chance to learn a little more about what you went through, and it'll be fun to see what options they come up with. Ask each of the guests to write down a comment about your child with or without her braces. Your potluck will be filled with interesting dishes, laughs, and a good time!

- **Relax.** What could be better than spending a couple of hours being pampered, or perhaps a round of golf or a trip to the beach? Not much! Take your child out—celebrate them making it through their treatment. They'll walk out feeling and looking great!

Doing some of these things, such as chewing gum, may still not be good for your child's teeth or their body overall. But doing it on a special occasion, and not making a habit out of it, won't cause any harm.

Of course, nobody can celebrate unless we started. There really is no time like the present.

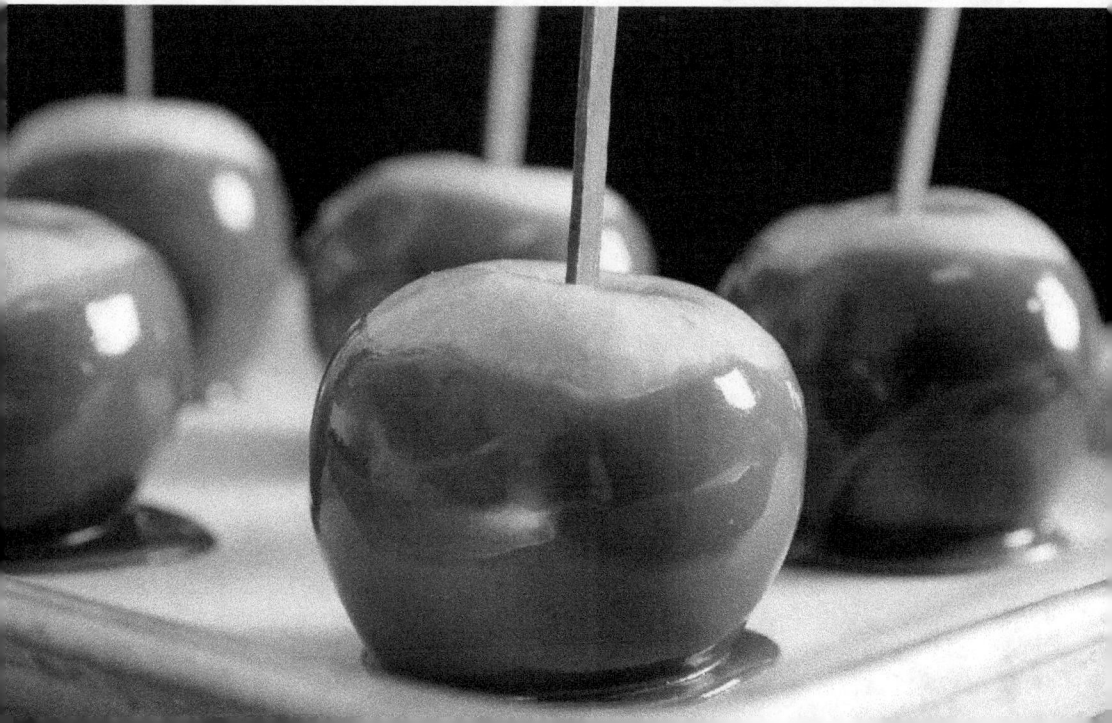

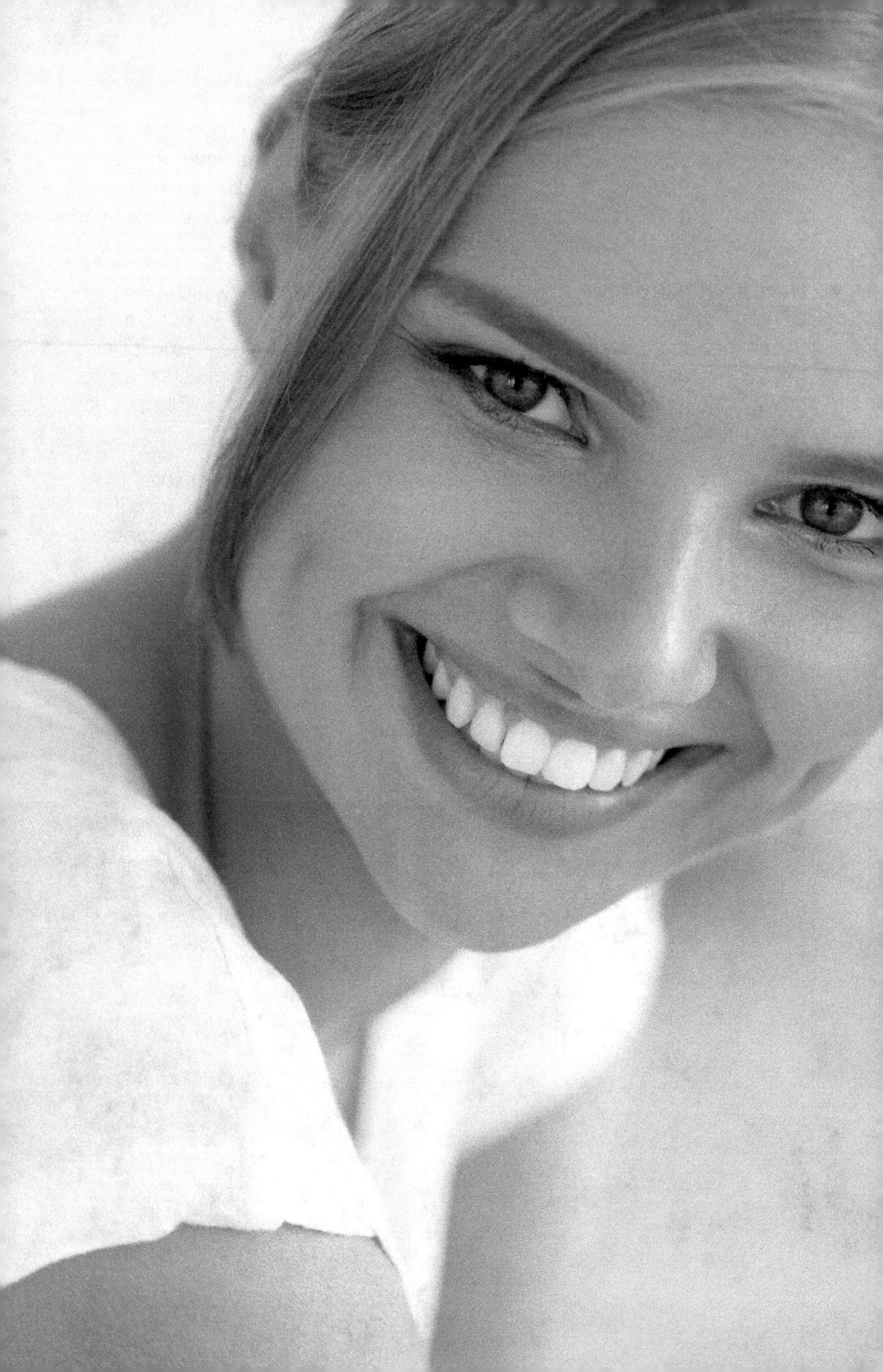

CHAPTER 12

What About My Smile?

Mom, Dad, I'm not going to kid you: if braces and/or orthodontic treatment was advised when you were eight or ten or twelve and, for whatever reason, it didn't happen, and you now have misaligned teeth, periodontal problems because of them, a smile you often hide, or jaw/TMJ pain, it may not be an easy fix. It may not even be fixable with orthodontics or braces. But often, to the surprise of adults, braces including invisible braces can do a significant amount of good for people thirty, forty, or even fifty years old. You may still be able to go from an embarrassing smile you often hide to a beautiful smile you love! You also may be able to enjoy better oral health, gently and gradually without having teeth pulled and without surgery. Many adults see ten years of age disappear from their faces!

The only way to know what the options are is with a complete, expert orthodontic exam.

At our office, we treat a lot of parents of patients, just like you, and a number of our adult patients come from referrals. You can arrange for your exam by speaking to any of the treatment coordinators at the office.

"After years of being told I needed surgery, my results are amazing without it. I'm finally able to smile in holiday photos." — Michael R.

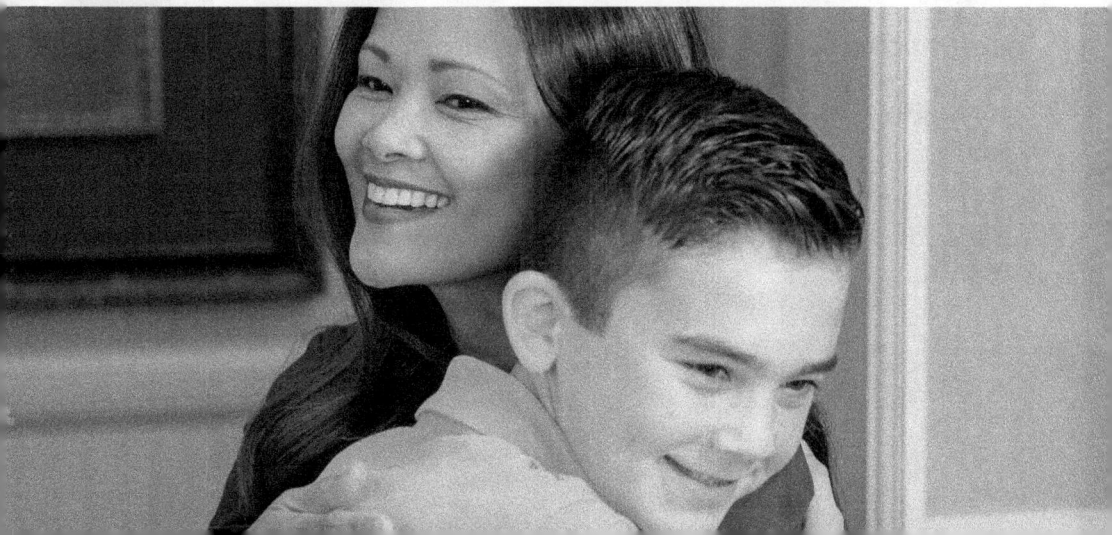

FAQS

Here is a handy resource guide of frequently asked questions and orthodontic terminology, many of which are answered throughout the book.

What might happen if your child's teeth or bite doesn't quite "fit"?
The fact is, the sooner you straighten your child's smile, the faster it will develop as it should: straight, clean, and healthy!

Who are some famous faces who've worn braces?
Gwen Stefani. Prince Harry. Drew Barrymore. Tom Cruise. Dakota Fanning. Danny Glover.

Can I see what my child's straight teeth might look like before the procedure is done?
Yes! With Invisalign treatment, the digital scan technology allows the doctor to show anticipated future bite and smile images.

Will I be able to afford my child's braces?
Not only are most orthodontic procedures cheaper than ever, but insurance, payment plans, and a variety of other financing options make braces more affordable than they've ever been.

Will getting braces be painful for my child?
Not anymore! Modern technology—and choosing the right orthodontist—can ensure that your child enjoys his/her orthodontic experience.

How much school will my child miss because of braces?
Not much, actually. After initial visits and, barring the actual procedure itself, most visits and/or adjustments are routine and can take anywhere from fifteen to forty-five minutes.

Is it really such a big deal if my child has crooked teeth?
Unfortunately, yes. Eroding, crooked, or unaligned smiles can take time to happen, but the time to act is now. Orthodontic irregularities don't just heal on their own or "go away" if you ignore them.

What are some of the warning signs that my child might need to go to the orthodontist?

There are many, but here are a few of the most common: early or late loss of teeth, protruding teeth, grinding or clenching of teeth, and speech difficulty.

What kind of "side effects" are caused by crooked teeth?

Some of the more frequent ones we see include headaches, toothaches, mouth breathing, chipped or worn down teeth, snoring, and drooling.

What makes an orthodontist more qualified than a dentist?

Orthodontists are dental specialists who have completed two to three years of additional education beyond dental school to learn the proper way to align teeth and jaws.

Why should I choose a specialist for my child's orthodontic care?

Unique treatment requirements and otherwise difficult bite problems are common, everyday scenarios for your orthodontist. In the interest of receiving the most efficient and effective orthodontic treatment possible, choose an orthodontic specialist.

How do I know if my doctor is an orthodontist?

Only orthodontists can belong to the American Association of Orthodontists (AAO).

What is a treatment coordinator?

During your initial consultation(s), you will usually be assigned a patient contact person—we call this person a "treatment coordinator" in our office— with whom to schedule appointments, confer with rescheduling and, of course, answer any and all questions you may have.

Why is early treatment so important?

Age seven is the earliest time your orthodontist can determine future jaw and tooth alignment. That's because, at the age of seven, your child's upper and lower permanent front teeth are developing. These teeth set the stage for future jaw position and serious problems can develop if they come into the wrong position.

Is there such a thing as a child being too old for braces?

There is no age that is "too old for braces" but some orthodontic issues are best treated at younger ages.

What if I don't believe in early orthodontics?

Well, you're entitled to your opinion, but this is like saying you don't believe in the sun. You can hide from it, pretend it's not there, or refuse to acknowledge it, but the simple fact remains. If you're not aware of the potential risks, you can get burnt.

Will my child actually need braces at seven?

Probably not. While we inform parents their child needs an initial exam at age seven, we also mention that most children will not need braces until eleven to thirteen years of age.

What is a crossbite?

A crossbite is a condition where a tooth is either closer to the cheek or the tongue than its opposing tooth. These can occur when the upper and lower teeth grow at different rates, or even when the lower jaw grows disproportionately with the upper jaw.

Where should I start to look for treatment if I'm concerned about my child's jaw development?

If you suspect your child might have a crossbite or other issues, approach your family dentist and ask about orthodontics.

Why should I address a crossbite?

Crossbites can lead to pain, discomfort, abnormal wear, asymmetric growth and lack of confidence as your child begins to feel insecure because of this very treatable problem.

What is Invisalign?

The Invisalign system is the virtually invisible way to straighten your teeth and achieve the dazzling smile you've always dreamed of. Using advanced 3-D computer-imaging technology, Invisalign depicts your complete treatment plan, from the initial position of your teeth to the final desired position.

What are the primary benefits of Invisalign?

Like the word that inspired them, Invisalign aligners are practically clear; or as close to "invisible" as one can get. No one may even notice you're wearing these virtually invisible braces, making Invisalign a seamless fit with your lifestyle and day-to-day interactions with others.

How do I get started with Invisalign?

It's simple: just make an appointment with your local orthodontist for an initial consultation. Most doctors will offer a free initial consultation to see if you are a good candidate for Invisalign.

How will Invisalign effectively move my teeth?

Aligners are the foundation for, and work in unison with, the Invisalign system. Like brackets and arch wires are to braces, Invisalign aligners move teeth by using the appropriate placement of controlled force on your child's teeth.

How many patients are being treated with Invisalign?

More than one million patients worldwide have been treated with Invisalign. The number of Invisalign smiles grows daily.

Is Invisalign appropriate for my child?

Possibly, yes. Invisalign now has a system designed specifically for teens!

How does Invisalign Teen work?

Aligners snap on your teeth easily. They are comfortable and practically invisible. Invisalign Teen allows permanent teeth to grow and gently and continuously moves your teeth in small increments. Aligners are worn for one or two weeks, then you swap them for a new pair.

Why are metal braces still so popular?

Metal braces are very strong and can withstand most types of treatment. Today's metal braces are smaller, sleeker, and more polished than ever before.

Are so-called "clear braces" effective?

Ceramic braces are very strong and generally do not stain. Adults like to choose ceramic braces because they "blend in" with the teeth and are less noticeable than metal. These are the types of braces actor Tom Cruise had.

Are clear braces appropriate for adults?
Absolutely! Adults of all ages can enjoy the same cosmetic and health benefits of properly aligned teeth with clear braces.

What are some of my payment options in addition to insurance?
One way many patients pay for their procedures is by utilizing the benefits of what is known as "flex spending," where their employer matches their spending commitment.

What if my child has a "braces emergency" before or after office hours?
If you are experiencing an orthodontic emergency that can't wait for regular office hours, most orthodontic offices have a special number to call, either before, during, or after business hours. If this information isn't given to you readily, ask how your doctor's office handles emergencies.

Can a salt water rinse help deal with irritation caused by braces?
Absolutely; warm saltwater rinses soothe the cheek lining, which can get aggravated by your child's braces.

How do I make a salt water rinse?
To make a salt water rinse, mix ½ teaspoon of table salt in one cup of warm water. Stir until the salt is completely dissolved. Gently swish about ¼ of the cup in your mouth for 30 seconds. Make sure you force the water over the areas that feel sore. Then spit the water into the sink. Repeat until the entire cup is gone.

What if my child plays sports and needs a mouth guard?
The best advice for patients or parents looking for a mouth guard can be obtained from your pediatrician, dentist, pediatric dentist, orthodontist or oral surgeon. All of these specialists are uniquely trained to offer customized advice in order to help you prevent a sports-related dental or facial injury.

What about brushing with braces?
Here are some simple tips you can share with your child for the best results when brushing with braces on:

• Brush your teeth in the morning, after you eat and before bed.

- Brush, rinse, and look; if you find any areas that are not clean, brush them again.

- Brush your gums as you brush your teeth (massage and stimulate).

- If no toothpaste is available, brush without.

- If you are unable to brush, rinse your mouth vigorously with water.

- Replace your old toothbrush every 3 months or when it gets worn out, whichever comes first.

- It is absolutely essential that you continue regular visits to your family dentist for checkups and cleanings throughout your orthodontic treatment!

What type of foods should my child avoid while wearing braces?

There are four main types of food your child should avoid while wearing braces: **hard foods,** like ice, popcorn, peanut brittle, rock candy, and corn on the cob; **sticky foods,** like caramels, bubble gum, taffy, and suckers; **chewy foods,** like pizza crust, crusty breads, beef jerky, and gummy bears; and **sugary foods and drinks,** like cake, ice cream, cookies, pie, candy, and soda pop.

Why are retainers so important?

As we age, teeth naturally shift to the middle and crowd. Combined with late growth of the lower jaw, shifting of the teeth is expected following orthodontic treatment. Therefore, retainers are extremely important in the maintenance of your new smile following orthodontic treatment.

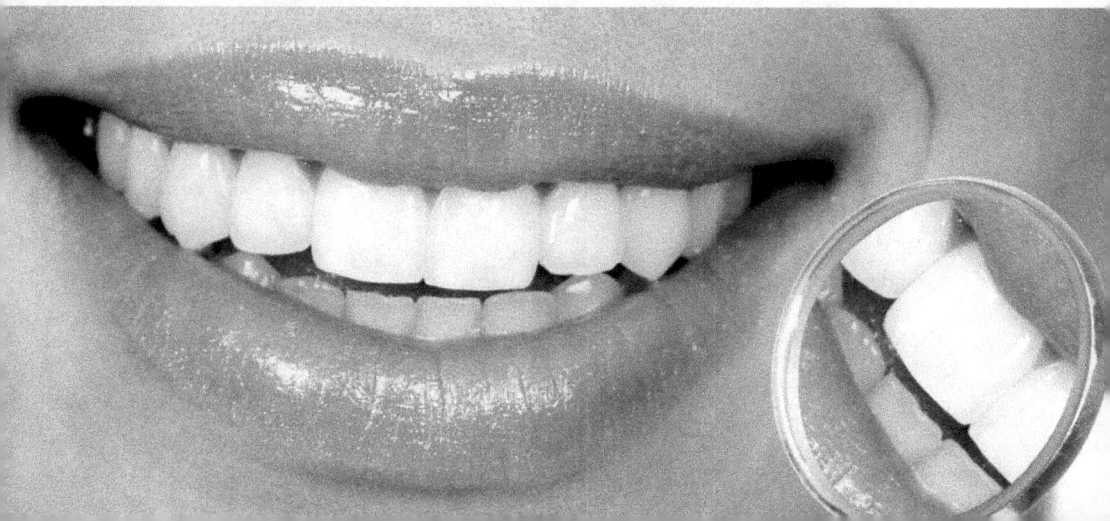

RESACES

Before or after your consultation, you may want more information for yourself or your son or daughter. The following website provides valuable insight to help you make the right decision for your child.

Braces.org is the "all about braces site" of the American Association of Orthodontists. This is the official regulatory body and professional association of orthodontists, and only orthodontists (not dentists) can be members. Here you will receive accurate, up-to-date information on orthodontics.

ABOUT THE AUTHORS

Dr. Brad Mokris

I often get asked how I ended up becoming an orthodontist. Well the truth is, it wasn't my first choice of career paths. In kindergarten, my teacher asked the class what we wanted to be when we grew up. Confidently, I stood up and told the class I wanted to be an astronaut. As I sat down, proud of my distinguished future profession, my best friend whispered in my ear: "sometimes when astronauts go up in space, they get lost and don't come back down." Needless to say, I never sent my application in to NASA. True story. I did, however, have the experience of getting braces in high school, and after getting them off, I spent many hours shadowing my orthodontist and other orthodontists throughout high school and college. I know everyone has an opinion of the "perfect" career. But for me, this was it. I am very proud and appreciative of what I get to do everyday. As an orthodontist, I create smiles... what a job!

After college and a not so brief hiatus surfing in Hawaii, I spent 7 years in Gainesville, Florida receiving my dental and orthodontic training. It was there that I met the one and only love of my life, Jennifer, also a dentist practicing in Fernandina Beach. We have 4 children, Avery, Reese, Austin and Graham. Our children are our life, and they keep us on our toes endlessly. But we do manage to travel quite a bit, whether its up to the Carolinas to see my parents and 3 brothers, or right down the road for an afternoon at the beautiful North Florida beaches. Orthodontics is a constantly evolving and exciting field. At Coastline Orthodontics, we truly believe we have an obligation to provide our patients with the safest and most advanced treatment options available. This is not something that is learned once but an ongoing learning process with continuing education and a lifelong pursuit to be the best at what we do. These aspirations help us to give our patients individualized treatment geared for the most healthy and efficient path towards a beautiful smile.

Degrees

- B.S. in Biology, 2003, University of North Carolina at Chapel Hill
- Doctor of Dental Medicine, 2008, University of Florida
- Master of Science/Orthodontic Certificate, 2011, University of Florida

Dental & Orthodontic Memberships

- American Dental Association
- Florida Dental Association

- Northeast District Dental Association
- Jacksonville Dental Society
- Florida Association of Orthodontists
- Southern Association of Orthodontists
- American Association of Orthodontists

Dr. Valerie Minor

I did not always want to be an orthodontist. I did consider dentistry or possibly medicine as a career choice after completing a 9th grade science project on "Which toothpaste whitens the best?" However, when it was time to go off to college, I could not imagine going to school for another 8+ years, so I decided to get an engineering degree. After graduating from North Carolina State University with degrees in Chemical Engineering and Pulp and Paper Science, I was fortunate to get a great job working for Rayonier in Fernandina Beach, FL, near my hometown.

After a short time working in the manufacturing industry, I decided that this was not for me. While working at Rayonier, I spent some time shadowing Dr. Suellen Rodeffer in her orthodontic practice. I realized very quickly that this was a profession that I would love. It seemed to combine the engineering that I had learned with the interaction and care for people that I was missing in a manufacturing facility. I was amazed to see the changes that could take place and the smiles on the faces of Dr. Rodeffer's patients when they would leave her office. At that time, Dr. Rodeffer joked with me that one day I would come back and be one of her partners. Little did I know that God was planning that very path for me.

With the blessing of my wonderful husband, I made up my mind to pursue that goal. After taking several prerequisite courses while still working for Rayonier, we packed up and moved to Gainesville, FL, for 7 years of training at the University of Florida. I am so blessed that God saw fit to lead me down this amazing journey. I joined Rodeffer and Garner Orthodontics in 2006, and my husband Will was able to teach and start the baseball program at the newly opened Yulee High School. We became Rodeffer, Garner, and Minor Orthodontics shortly thereafter, and now we have changed the name again to Coastline Orthodontics with the addition of Dr. Mokris to our practice. My husband, Will is part owner of Netting Professionals, a business that specializes in sports netting and supplies for recreational leagues, high schools, colleges, and pro sports teams. We have 4 amazing children named Harper, Savannah, Ava, and Addison (twins). Needless to say, our kids keep us very busy, but they are the joy of our lives.

When I am not at the office or at one of our children's activities, I enjoy going to the beach, exercising, reading, and watching sporting events – especially Gator football and baseball. I am so blessed to be an orthodontist, in such a beautiful area with amazing people. I enjoy getting to know our patients and watching the transformation that takes place as they develop more confidence in their smiles. We hope that you will feel comfortable in our practice, and we appreciate the trust that you have placed in us to take care of your smile.

Degrees

- Chemical Engineering and Pulp and Paper Science, 1997, North Carolina State University
- Doctor of Dental Medicine, 2003, University of Florida
- Master of Science/Orthodontic Certificate, 2006 University of Florida

Dental & Orthodontic Memberships

- American Dental Association
- Florida Dental Association
- Northeast District Dental Association
- Jacksonville Dental Society
- Florida Association of Orthodontists
- Southern Association of Orthodontists
- American Association of Orthodontists

THE NEXT STEP:

Your Customized Smile Analysis

When you are ready, I urge you to schedule your **Customized Smile Analysis**, with a complimentary consultation; safe, digital x-rays (a $249 value) and exam; and report to you and your son or daughter—all without cost or obligation.

Call us at 904.600.4749 or go to www.coastlineorthodontics.com to schedule your own Customized Smile Analysis.

www.ingramcontent.com/pod-product-compliance
Lightning Source LLC
Chambersburg PA
CBHW070814280326
41934CB00012B/3186